# KEYS TO PARENTING A CHILD WITH CEREBRAL PALSY

Jane Faulkner Leonard, P.T., M.S.H.P.
Sherri L. Cadenhead, M.S.P.T., P.C.S.
Margaret E. Myers, O.T.R.

RISE Library
618.92
LEO

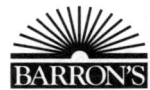

*Cover photo by Paul Vincent Kuntz, Texas Children's Hospital*

Photos on pages 39, 59, 91, 97, 143, and 173 by Paul Vincent Kuntz and James deLeon, Texas Children's Hospital

**DEDICATION**
To my parents, Jim and Judy Faulkner, who lovingly and skillfully raised their little girl with cerebral palsy. They are the source of all that I believe about myself and God's gift in my life.
*Jane Faulkner Leonard, P.T., M.S.H.P.*

To my exceptional friends, the Fishers and the Stumpfs, to my mentors at the University of Oklahoma, and to the children who inspire me and give my life meaning.
*Sherri Cadenhead, M.S.P.T., P.C.S.*

To all the children and parents I have had the honor to work with who have been my teachers and have helped me learn what it means to have hope, determination, and perseverance.
*Margaret Myers, O.T.R.*

© Copyright 1997 by Barron's Educational Series, Inc.

All rights reserved.
No part of this book may be reproduced in any form, by photostat, microfilm, xerography, or any other means, or incorporated into any information retrieval system, electronic or mechanical, without the written permission of the copyright owner.

*All inquiries should be addressed to:*
Barron's Educational Series, Inc.
250 Wireless Boulevard
Hauppauge, New York 11788

Library of Congress Catalog Card No. 97-12492
International Standard Book No. 0-7641-0091-2

**Library of Congress Cataloging-in-Publication Data**
Leonard, Jane Faulkner.
    Keys to parenting a child with cerebral palsy / Jane Faulkner Leonard, Sherri Cadenhead, Margaret Myers.
       p. cm. — (Barron's parenting keys)
    Includes bibliographical references and index.
    ISBN 0-7641-0091-2
    1. Cerebral palsied children—Family relations. 2. Cerebral palsied children—Home care. 3. Parent and child. I. Cadenhead, Sherri. II. Myers, Margaret, O.T.R. III. Title. IV. Series.
RJ496.C4L385    1997
618.92'836—DC21                                      97-12492
                                                                                 CIP

PRINTED IN THE UNITED STATES OF AMERICA
987654321

# CONTENTS

Introduction     vi

**Part One—Understanding Cerebral Palsy**     1
1. What Are Babies with Cerebral Palsy Like?     2
2. What Is Cerebral Palsy?     5
3. Types of Cerebral Palsy     8
4. Reasons to Learn More     11
5. Common Misunderstandings     13

**Part Two—Adjusting to Your Child with Cerebral Palsy**     18
6. Sorting Out Your Emotions     19
7. Relating to Family, Friends, and Strangers     23
8. Getting to Know Other Parents     26
9. Counseling and Professional Support     28

**Part Three—Balancing Family Relationships**     30
10. Everyone in Your Family Is Special     31
11. You and Your Spouse     34
12. Brothers and Sisters     37
13. Grandparents     42
14. Respite Care and Day Care     44
15. Should We Have Another Baby?     47
16. Single-Parent Family Concerns     49

**Part Four—Your Child's Total Well-Being**     52
17. What Is Normal Development?     53
18. Your Child's Physical Development     56
19. Your Child's Mental Development     61
20. Your Child's Social Development     65
21. Common Health Problems     68
22. Vision, Hearing, and Dental Concerns     72

| 23 | Helping Your Child to Eat | 74 |
| 24 | Working with Your Child's Healthcare Team | 77 |
| 25 | What Is Therapy? | 80 |
| 26 | New Trends in Medical Management | 83 |

## Part Five—Raising a Child with Cerebral Palsy — 87
| 27 | What Can We Expect? | 88 |
| 28 | Getting Organized | 92 |
| 29 | Teaching Your Child to Play | 96 |
| 30 | Helping Your Child Become Independent | 99 |
| 31 | Home Care and Habilitation Training | 102 |
| 32 | Managing Behavior and Discipline | 104 |

## Part Six—Your Child's Learning — 108
| 33 | Your Child's Right to Education: It's the Law | 109 |
| 34 | Your Rights as a Parent | 112 |
| 35 | Comprehensive Evaluations | 115 |
| 36 | What Is Early Intervention? | 117 |
| 37 | Regular and Special Education | 121 |
| 38 | Training Plans: IFSP, IEP, and IHP | 124 |
| 39 | Working with Your Child's Education Team | 128 |
| 40 | What Are Mainstreaming and Inclusion? | 130 |
| 41 | Helping Your Child Learn | 133 |
| 42 | Helping Your Child Communicate | 136 |
| 43 | What Is Assistive Technology? | 140 |

## Part Seven—Your Child's Future — 144
| 44 | Your Child Can Make Friends | 145 |
| 45 | Developing Your Child's Interests | 148 |
| 46 | Developing Realistic Goals | 151 |
| 47 | Making a Positive Contribution to Society | 154 |
| 48 | Transition: Planning for the Next Step | 157 |
| 49 | Going to Work | 159 |
| 50 | Handling Sex Education | 163 |
| 51 | Sexuality, Marriage, and Parenthood | 167 |
| 52 | Places to Live | 171 |
| 53 | Meeting Your Financial Needs | 175 |

| 54 | Financial Planning and Guardianship | 179 |
| 55 | Letting Go | 182 |

| Questions and Answers | 184 |
|---|---|
| Glossary | 186 |
| Appendix | |
|     Tips for Positioning Your Child | 192 |
|     Suggested Reading | 194 |
|     Resources | 198 |
|     Assistive Technology Resources | 205 |
| Index | 211 |

# INTRODUCTION

**How Do You Feel?**

For some families, just opening a book with the words *cerebral palsy* in the title may be an overwhelming experience. That is a very natural reaction. Just keep this book on your bedside table, and when you are ready, read a little bit at a time.

Some families may feel a tremendous sense of relief after being given a name for their child's problem. Often, mothers, fathers, and grandparents have had an eerie feeling that something was not right. This baby just did not feel or move the way your other child moved or develop the way your friend's or sister's babies developed.

Perhaps throughout your pregnancy, delivery, and lengthy hospital stay, you have already won a battle for your precious baby's life. You are to be congratulated, but you feel exhausted.

You may feel angry or confused because you have taken this baby to one or several professionals and received no answers about why your baby is different. Your baby may have had problems nursing at the breast or bottle. He felt unnaturally stiff or, more commonly, very floppy. Often, this baby has failed to hold his head up, roll over, or sit by himself. Many times the medical professionals have wisely said, "Let's wait and see awhile. No two babies are alike, and many normal babies develop at different rates." Still, you feel lost.

Perhaps you have felt as if no one was listening to you, and no one was taking your child's health and movement problems seriously. You may have been described by friends, family, or members of the medical community as nervous, inexperienced, anxious, or demanding in your role as a parent.

Your normally healthy infant may have become very sick, had an unexpected seizure, or had a head injury. Now, your baby is not doing things that he was doing before. He is no longer developing like he should.

For every set of parents of a child with cerebral palsy, a day arrives when a doctor sits down and discusses the possibility that your child may have cerebral palsy. Your doctor will reassure you that the damage your child's brain has received will not worsen over time. The doctor will advise you that your son or daughter may require special medical care, long-term therapy, and a carefully designed educational program to reach his or her highest potential.

On that day, we hope you receive this book. It should serve as an introductory guidebook to provide the information, resources, and options to assist you now and over time. *Keys to Parenting a Child with Cerebral Palsy* is written in short chapters called Keys. Within each Key, you will find information and suggestions to help you raise your child. Each of the seven major parts of the book are introduced by a summary that describes the contents of that section.

You are beginning a special journey. This journey will slowly change you as a person, as a parent, and as a family with a child who has special needs. Life experiences that lead to personal growth are often difficult. You can, at times, expect to feel very, very frustrated and ready to give up. Use this book as a starting point to build yourself, your child, and your family a strong and supportive home and community network.

**Who Are the Authors?**

Jane Faulkner Leonard, P.T., M.S.H.P., is a physical therapist at Texas Children's Hospital in Houston, Texas. For 13 years she has worked with infants, children, and young adults with cerebral palsy. She is certified in the neurodevelopmental treatment approach for children with cerebral palsy. As a result of a premature birth in 1961, Ms. Leonard has cerebral palsy and spent much of her childhood with braces and crutches. She faced firsthand many of the challenges your child may face. She credits her parents' guidance with steering her toward fully independent adulthood, including college, employment, marriage, and motherhood.

Sherri L. Cadenhead, M.S.P.T., P.C.S., is also a physical therapist. She has worked with children and adults with cerebral palsy for seven years and has earned her advanced master's degree and board certification in pediatric physical therapy. She gained valuable experience while working in a facility in Oklahoma for people with developmental disabilities. Currently, Ms. Cadenhead coordinates the Texas Children's Hospital Seating and Mobility Clinic and has provided training for staff caring for children with cerebral palsy in Mexico.

Margaret E. Myers, O.T.R., is an occupational therapist who has worked in pediatrics for the past five years in neonatal intensive care units, outpatient departments, and schools. She has experience working with children who have a wide variety of disabilities including cerebral palsy. Ms. Myers has expertise in feeding and developmental therapy. She is currently at home with her one-year-old daughter learning the true meaning of the word "Mommy."

**Acknowledgments**

With appreciation and special thanks to our colleagues, patients, and parents at Texas Children's Hospital Department of Physical Medicine and Rehabilitation, without whom the opportunity to write this book would not have been possible. And to Reyna, Karen, Patricia, and Vanessa who patiently helped produce this manuscript.

# PART ONE

# UNDERSTANDING CEREBRAL PALSY

You have learned that your child has cerebral palsy, but what does that mean? Part One of this book describes the ways in which children with cerebral palsy are similar to each other. This information may be helpful to parents who are unsure about their child's diagnosis. In this part, you will find an understandable definition of cerebral palsy. The different causes and types of cerebral palsy are described, as well.

In Part One, you will learn why it is so very important for you to discover as much as you can about your child's condition. Through knowledge you can advocate for your child. In this part, also, the myths and misunderstandings about cerebral palsy are put to rest.

# 1

# WHAT ARE BABIES WITH CEREBRAL PALSY LIKE?

Many parents and families, when first told their child has cerebral palsy, desperately want to know what babies with cerebral palsy are like. They frequently take their baby to many different professionals hoping that someone can answer their questions with certainty. What will this child be like when she's an adult? Will she be able to walk? Will she be able to speak? Will she be able to live independently? Will she look normal? Will she live? Can I take care of her at home?

Children with cerebral palsy have only one thing in common. They have all experienced some sort of brain damage. The brain damage does not worsen as the child grows older, but it does cause permanent problems with movement. Sometimes speaking, swallowing, seeing, hearing, or thinking can be affected.

There are tremendous differences in the way babies with cerebral palsy will look, move, function, and behave. However, families report a group of common problems that occur more frequently in children with cerebral palsy. Your child may show one or several of these characteristics. Some of these symptoms develop slowly over time while others may be apparent very early in the infant's life. Feeding problems, in particular, may be evident immediately after birth.

## Movement Problems

A child with cerebral palsy *always* has problems with voluntary or purposeful movement. She may have difficulty lifting or holding up her head. She may lay quite still in her crib with parents waiting and watching for her to lift her head or push up on her arms. She may not roll. Instead, she may arch her back and move backward on the mattress with most of her weight on the back of her head. Often, the child will break her hair and develop a bald spot on the back of her head as a result of frequently arching backward.

When held in your arms, the baby may slump into your shoulder or drape limply across your back. You may consciously or unconsciously position your arms to support her back, neck, and head for a much longer period than you would with another infant. On the other hand, your baby may be unnaturally stiff when she is held. It may be difficult to bend her at the hips. She may strongly arch her head, neck, and back. Her legs may feel very stiff and straight, and very often cross each other like a pair of scissors. It may be difficult to open and spread her legs for diapering. Her hands may stay in a tight fist with her thumbs tucked tightly inside. Her toes may also remain tightly curled.

Your child may be limp at rest and become stiff when she tries to move. After moving, she may collapse again, like a floppy Raggedy Ann doll. In general, your child will learn movement skills slowly. When she performs a movement skill such as sitting, standing, or walking, she will often do it in an unusual way.

## Feeding Problems

A child with cerebral palsy often has difficulty feeding. She may suck weakly and have difficulty coordinating mouth and throat muscles for efficient and safe eating. Eating may be tiresome and take a long time. Occasionally, a child may need special feeding methods or equipment to keep her safe and growing well. Your child with cerebral palsy may have no feeding problems at all and, in time, will eat regular table food with ordinary or special utensils. If needed, therapy can be very helpful in improving feeding skills.

## Problems with Being Calm, Awake, and Alert

Babies with cerebral palsy often have personalities and behaviors that are identical to any normal infant. They all cry, sleep, and need to be held and cuddled. They need their parents to help them explore the people and objects in their world.

Infants with cerebral palsy are more likely to have difficulty being calm or staying alert. Some are irritable or jittery and have longer crying episodes than those experienced by infants who just have colic. Crying may be accompanied by stiffness, arching, or unusual trembling. Crying, trembling, and jitteriness are normal to some degree in *all* babies; however, in infants with cerebral palsy, they may last longer, be more extreme, and will *always* be coupled with movement problems.

Other babies with cerebral palsy are average or very easy babies in terms of behavior. They may sleep a great deal of the time. Some must always be awakened for feeding. They do not remain alert for very long. Often, these babies are limp or floppy. They tend to stay in whatever position you leave them in. They may fail to focus their eyes on faces or objects and may not turn their heads to respond to sounds. They may be easily startled by sudden movements or loud sounds that other babies become used to over time. This is related to the movement problems and not nervousness.

Although no two babies are alike, babies with cerebral palsy have some things in common. Your child's doctor will ask questions about these similarities, feel the baby, and watch her move. The doctor will ask questions about feeding, temperament, and other things. This information and the results of medical tests will be taken into consideration before your child is given a diagnosis of cerebral palsy.

# 2

# WHAT IS CEREBRAL PALSY?

Cerebral palsy is a disorder in which the brain is damaged, resulting in abnormal posture and movement. The brain damage is permanent, but it does not worsen as the child grows older. Cerebral palsy does not have a cure, and a child will not grow out of it. However, many children with cerebral palsy improve with excellent care and therapy.

*Cerebral* comes from the Latin word meaning brain. *Palsy* refers to lack of muscle control. Cerebral palsy is sometimes called static encephalopathy. *Static* means the brain damage is permanent and does not worsen over time. Encephalopathy comes from the term *encephalo-* meaning brain and *-pathy* which is a problem or an abnormal condition. As a result of the brain damage, the brain sends incorrect signals to the child's muscles, resulting in abnormal movement patterns.

Cerebral palsy usually occurs before, during, or shortly after birth. The developing brain is more at risk for damage during pregnancy, labor, delivery, and the initial days of early life. The abnormal movement symptoms of cerebral palsy can also be acquired later in life if the brain is damaged by infection or injury. Doctors will usually diagnose cerebral palsy only if the brain damage occurred before one year of age.

Half-a-million Americans have cerebral palsy. It can be a very mild condition such as a slight limp or stiffness while walking. It can be severe, resulting in complete inability to control body movements. Each year, approximately 3,000 babies are born with cerebral palsy. Approximately 1,000 young children will acquire it or similar conditions each year as a result of accidents or illnesses.

## Causes of Cerebral Palsy

Cerebral palsy can be caused by *lack of oxygen* or *blood circulation to the brain* before, during, or after birth. This can occur for many reasons including loss of the baby's heartbeat, umbilical cord wrapped tightly around the baby's neck, separation of the placenta from the wall of the uterus, a drop or rise in the mother's or infant's blood pressure, failure of the baby to breathe well after delivery, secretions in the baby's airway, or breathing and blood supply problems in the infant or child.

Cerebral palsy can also be caused by *bleeding* or *lack of adequate blood flow in the baby's brain.* Babies born prematurely are much more likely to have abnormal bleeding or hemorrhages in the brain. This often occurs in the areas of the brain called ventricles where cerebral spinal fluid circulates. Additionally, if the baby has abnormal blood vessels in the brain or if blockage occurs in a blood vessel that supplies the brain, cerebral palsy may result.

Cerebral palsy may occur if the baby's *brain structures did not develop completely or normally.* Lack of brain growth may result in small head size. This is called *microcephaly* or *small brain.* Physicians or nurses may measure a baby's head size before birth and after birth to check to see if the brain is growing as expected. Some babies have abnormal or missing brain structures, such as agenesis of corpus collosum, that may result in cerebral palsy.

Cerebral palsy may occur if the mother or baby have an *infection that harms the child's brain* before, during, or after birth. Examples include rubella or German measles during pregnancy, cytomegalovirus during pregnancy, herpes during pregnancy or delivery, and meningitis or encephalitis in infancy or childhood. Any viral, fungal, or bacterial infection that attacks the child's brain can result in the symptoms of cerebral palsy.

*Rh incompatibility*, if untreated, can cause cerebral palsy. Rh incompatibility occurs when a mother's immune system attacks her baby's tissue. This happens if her baby has a particular blood protein that the mother lacks. Through prenatal testing, this problem can be discovered and treated with medication to the mother and/or blood transfusions for the baby.

Cerebral palsy can be acquired through *accidents* that result in brain damage. Head injuries suffered during falls, motor vehicle collisions, and child abuse can cause cerebral palsy. Other accidental causes include poisoning, drowning, suffocation, or electrocution. Hypothermia or hyperthermia, an extremely low or extremely high body temperature, can cause brain damage that results in the symptoms of cerebral palsy.

Genetic disorders sometimes cause damage to the brain that can give a child the symptoms of cerebral palsy. Genetic disorders can be inherited by children from the parents. Cerebral palsy is *not* an inherited disorder. However, a child can have a movement disorder with symptoms that are similar to cerebral palsy if he has inherited a genetic disorder.

Complications in pregnancy, labor, and delivery can sometimes increase the likelihood that a child will have brain damage. An unusually long or short labor, delivery by forceps, a breech presentation, premature labor, or multiple births such as twins, triplets, and quadruplets can increase the risk for cerebral palsy. In some cases, one twin can have cerebral palsy and the other twin not. Sometimes, both twins will have cerebral palsy.

Unfortunately, sometimes the cause of cerebral palsy cannot be found. A child may have the characteristics of cerebral palsy, but medical testing may not show a cause. Most cases of cerebral palsy happen for unknown reasons or because of the above-mentioned prenatal factors. Ask your child's doctor to show you diagrams, CT scans, or MRIs of your child's brain to help you better understand his condition.

# 3

# TYPES OF CEREBRAL PALSY

Your child's movement problems may be described as one or more types of cerebral palsy. The type of cerebral palsy is a description of the way your child's body responds when he tries to move or you try to move him. The type of cerebral palsy depends on what area or areas in your child's brain are damaged.

**What Are the Five Basic Types of Cerebral Palsy?**

*Spastic*

Spastic cerebral palsy typically occurs when the motor cortex or corticospinal tracts of the brain are damaged. The terms *spasticity* and *hypertonia* are often used to describe this condition. A child with spastic cerebral palsy has one or more limbs that feel stiff and are difficult to move smoothly. He may be described as tight and may often hold a spastic body part in an unusual position. For example, it may be easy for your child to bend his knee but difficult for him to straighten it. He may tend to use a spastic body part less often than a normal body part. If he wants to use his hand, he frequently will move his whole arm in an unusual pattern.

*Athetoid*

The child with athetoid cerebral palsy alternates between being stiff and floppy. He often stiffens or arches backward when he is moved suddenly or becomes excited, and then he collapses. Sometimes, he is so tight and stiff that you can barely bend him. Seconds later, he is so floppy that he cannot hold his head or body up. The child with athetoid cerebral palsy frequently has damage to the basal ganglia area of the brain. Athetosis is also referred to as *dyskinesia* or *dystonia*.

*Ataxic*

The child with ataxic cerebral palsy frequently has tremors or trembling when he tries to move. His head and trunk can tremor when he attempts to sit up, walk, or support himself. Sometimes, the more a child struggles with a posture or movement the greater the trembling becomes. This child may have poor coordination and tend to fear falling. When reaching for a toy, he may overshoot or undershoot a target. Ataxia is the result of damage to the cerebellum at the base of the brain.

*Hypotonic*

Hypotonia may occur because of damage throughout the whole brain. It usually is not possible to locate one specific area of damage. A child with hypotonic or low-toned cerebral palsy may be floppy all the time. He may feel soft and mushy when you hold him. He may be very flexible and appear to be double jointed. He may have difficulty holding his head up, rolling, sitting, creeping, or walking. He may tire quickly and often appear to be lazy or sleepy. He may often stay very still and will not try to move. The child with hypotonia may be described as a very happy baby who does not make many demands.

*Mixed*

Many children with cerebral palsy have more than one type. It is common for a child to be spastic but with a hypotonic trunk, or to be both spastic and athetoid. If several areas of the brain are damaged, then several types of cerebral palsy may be seen in combination in one child.

## What Parts of My Child's Body Are Affected?

In most cases of cerebral palsy, the muscles of the trunk (shoulders, back, hips, chest, and abdomen) are not as strong, as well-coordinated, or as balanced as in a child without cerebral palsy. However, children with cerebral palsy are frequently labeled by the problems that are observed in the arms or legs.

*Monoplegia*
Only one body part is affected. Monoplegia is uncommon.

*Diplegia*
Typically, both legs, the pelvis, and the hip muscles are more affected than the upper body. One side may be more severely affected than the other. This is a common pattern of cerebral palsy for premature babies. The arms are often involved in people with diplegia, but the legs are more severely affected than the arms.

*Hemiplegia*
An arm and leg on the same side of the body are most severely affected. Typically, the hand is more severely affected than the foot. For example, the child with hemiplegia can often walk without a crutch or cane but may have little functional use of the affected hand.

*Quadriplegia*
In quadriplegia, both arms, both legs, and the trunk are affected. Typically, the arms are somewhat more affected than the legs. All four limbs are sometimes affected equally. Often, one side of the body is more involved than the other.

No two children with cerebral palsy are truly alike. These classifications only help organize the treatment approach for a child with cerebral palsy. Each child's strengths and challenges are unique and individual. No other child is exactly like yours.

# 4

# REASONS TO LEARN MORE

It is important to ask questions about your child and to understand the answers given. Investigate programs, ideas, and treatments, now and in the future. As a parent or caregiver of a child with cerebral palsy, you need to be informed for several very important reasons.

No two children with cerebral palsy are alike. A parent must help design a unique life plan that balances a child's and family's individual medical, therapeutic, educational, vocational, social, and financial needs. Parents are partners in planning. Parents exercise, position, feed, discipline, teach, and communicate with their child daily. You know your child better than anyone, but it helps to learn all that you can.

No single surgery, medicine, or therapy can correct all of the problems caused by cerebral palsy; therefore, information is very important.

New possibilities are being developed for helping your child with cerebral palsy. An informed parent can help explore all the possibilities. New options include changed uses of medications that improve the ability to use muscles, new surgeries that improve function, and new types of therapy. New opportunities exist for children and adults to be educated, work, and live on their own.

Parents need to be informed because they have an important role as advocate for their child. An advocate helps keep the health care and education teams and the community focused on what is best for your child. The parent often provides a voice for the child if she cannot easily communicate her wants and needs.

You also need to gather resources for your child and family. These can help solve problems with money, answer questions about education, and much more. Knowing that resources are available will give you some piece of mind.

Having access to the latest information is one of the ways parents help their child to progress. By arming yourself with the latest up-to-date information, you can help your child do her very best.

# 5

# COMMON MISUNDERSTANDINGS

Cerebral palsy has been around for centuries. Many people have incorrect and outdated opinions about this common childhood disability. Hearing these myths can be upsetting and confusing. This key sheds light on this often misunderstood condition.

**Myth: Cerebral palsy is always inherited.**

**Fact:** Most common causes of cerebral palsy, including premature birth, infection, birth complications, and head injuries, are *not* inherited and thus are *not likely* to be repeated in future pregnancies. You should feel free to ask your physician if genetic testing might be helpful.

Genetic causes for movement problems that are similar to cerebral palsy are more likely if you have a family member with similar disabilities, family members intermarry, the child has multiple organ problems, or the child has an unusual appearance or physical features. If your child is diagnosed with cerebral palsy but some of these risk factors are present, you need genetic counseling. Unusual features sometimes noted in children with inherited disorders include

- unusual head size (small or large)
- unusual size, shape, or position of ears
- abnormalities in the fingers or toes (extra toes or fingers, missing toes or fingers, short stubby broad fingers)

- low hairline or unusual distribution of facial or body hair
- abnormal bone structure of face (wide or close set eyes, small bridge of nose)
- unusual condition of teeth (poor enamel, cone- or peg-shaped teeth).

**Myth: All children with cerebral palsy are mentally retarded.**

**Fact:** Between 50 percent and 75 percent of children with cerebral palsy have either some degree of mental retardation or learning disabilities. Many children with cerebral palsy have normal or even above normal intelligence, and their problems only involve their ability to move. Often, it is very difficult to test the intelligence of children with cerebral palsy because they may have difficulty speaking or using their hands.

Some children have severe or profound mental retardation. These children usually do not consistently respond to people, toys, or activities occurring near them. Other children have moderate retardation where learning new skills is a very slow process that requires intensive education and therapy. Many children with moderate retardation can be eventually taught to communicate, to use a special computer, or to read although usually significantly below expected grade level. Children with mild mental retardation or learning disabilities may require special education classes. Often, however, they can hold jobs in the community after special job coaching or training.

**Myth: All children with cerebral palsy are the same.**

**Fact:** The only thing that children with cerebral palsy have in common is that they all have brain damage and movement problems. The children can be quite different from one another depending on the extent and the location of brain damage. Some people with cerebral palsy will always need help with everything, while others hold jobs, marry, and become parents.

**Myth: Children with cerebral palsy do not improve.**

**Fact:** Almost all children with cerebral palsy will improve with appropriate education and therapy. Some children will improve only a little; however, it is still *very* important to seek appropriate education and ongoing therapy for these children in order to prevent complications and deformities. Other children improve dramatically with therapy and education. With training, most children will slowly improve over a very long period of time.

**Myth: Children with cerebral palsy do not need to attend school.**

**Fact:** Every effort should be made to keep your child attending school. Many special education services and therapy services are provided in school. If your child is ill or medically fragile, your child should still have a home-based, hospital-based, or special school program. Contact the special education department of your local school district to obtain information.

**Myth: Children with cerebral palsy are too difficult to care for at home. Most live in special residential or nursing homes.**

**Fact:** Most children with cerebral palsy live at home with their families and attend public school. Even children with complex medical needs like feeding tubes, tracheostomies, and ventilators are cared for at home with home health nurses assisting parents as needed.

**Myth: Children with cerebral palsy do not understand what is going on around them.**

**Fact:** It is important to realize that even if a child cannot talk, it is very possible that he can understand what is said. Many parents report that their children with cerebral palsy smile, laugh, or vocalize when they hear their mom or dad enter a room. Older children who are severely disabled have been reported to laugh at jokes or recognize songs on the radio or television commercials. Many children follow commands to hold a toy, eat a cracker, or go potty on the toilet. These abilities depend on the child's movement and thinking skills. Family and friends should speak in an age-appropriate, normal manner to both children and adults with cerebral palsy. This shows respect and provides an appropriate speech model for a child learning to communicate.

**Myth: Children with cerebral palsy do not feel pain.**

**Fact:** Children with cerebral palsy are capable of feeling both emotional and physical pain. Children who cannot speak have been reported to cry with tears running down their cheeks. This occurs if they are frightened or upset by being told of an impending doctor's visit for a blood test, hearing their loved ones have an argument, or other experiences.

Children with cerebral palsy and nondisabled children feel physical pain identically. Pain impulses are largely received by the spinal cord. Children with cerebral palsy have a normal spinal cord and thus feel pain like any other child. Proper anesthesia should be carefully administered to these children for surgeries and painful medical procedures.

**Myth: Children with severe cerebral palsy do not recognize their family members, so it does not matter who takes care of them.**

**Fact:** Even children with very severe disabilities often smile, coo, or make eye contact when being cared for by familiar, loving caretakers. They can become very stressed when left with people who are unfamiliar or when handled by anyone who is rough, highstrung, or abusive. Children who cannot talk sometimes show their stress through long periods of crying, sweating, flushed or pale skin, hiccups, vomiting, shaking, or unstable heart rate.

**Myth: If your child has cerebral palsy, the doctor or hospital must have done something wrong.**

**Fact:** In the majority of cases of cerebral palsy, your doctor or hospital could have done nothing differently to prevent your child's disability. Infections or viral illness early in a pregnancy are difficult or impossible to detect. Some birth complications happen unexpectedly with little or no warning. Cerebral palsy often happens in the first few hours or days of a newborn's life as a result of infection, prematurity, or bleeding in the brain. In most cases, your child's disability could not have been prevented by your physician or hospital.

# COMMON MISUNDERSTANDINGS

**Myth: If your child has cerebral palsy, you must have done something wrong.**

**Fact:** Cerebral palsy is most frequently caused by factors over which parents have little or no control. Many of the causes of cerebral palsy are not detectable by lab tests or ultrasounds during pregnancy. Viral infection in the mother during early pregnancy can be devastating to a baby's developing brain. Sometimes the mother may not even know she is sick. Even if the mother knows she has a viral illness while pregnant, the doctor usually cannot give her medicine to protect her baby from infection. Premature births are difficult to control or prevent. Except in cases of drug abuse or failure to receive prenatal care, the mother can usually do nothing to prevent cerebral palsy.

Myths and misunderstandings about children with cerebral palsy are common. Now you are armed with information that will help you understand your child better. This will help you to educate your community.

# PART TWO

# ADJUSTING TO YOUR CHILD WITH CEREBRAL PALSY

Part Two helps parents understand the many emotions they face having a child with cerebral palsy. You will find suggestions for dealing with these feelings and those of family, friends, and others. Using counseling for emotional support is discussed. Parents are encouraged to seek out other parents of children with disabilities. This could potentially help you the most in adjusting to your child.

# 6

# SORTING OUT YOUR EMOTIONS

Finding out that your child has cerebral palsy is one of the toughest emotional challenges that any family will ever face. Family members move through many painful and difficult emotions. Often, family members are in different stages of the adjustment process. It is *very* helpful to examine in detail the most common emotions felt by families of children with cerebral palsy.

**Feeling Overwhelmed and Confused**

Feeling overwhelmed and confused is a very common first reaction to being told that a child has cerebral palsy. Parents report feeling numb. It is very difficult to understand what the doctors, nurses, and therapists are trying to tell you. You feel as if you cannot concentrate. It is common to feel panicky or that you cannot take any more. Many parents complain that the healthcare team confuses them. When you feel overwhelmed, be patient and look for a support person who can help you. A support person can assist you by attending medical appointments, by helping you think through information, and by helping you make decisions. A social worker, counselor, clergyman, friend, or relative can often help. Sometimes, your spouse, who is also grieving, will have difficulty handling your feelings and needs at this time.

**Feeling Denial**

Denial is a way of thinking that protects your mind when a situation is *very, very* painful. Parents in denial constantly tell themselves and others that nothing serious or permanent is wrong with their child. A parent in denial can easily say that a one-year-old child who cannot lift her head up off the crib mattress will walk by herself very soon. Parents in denial often think that tests of their child's movement, speech, or thinking skills are wrong. They think that their child will magically become completely normal or close to normal in the near future.

Denial is a very common feeling. Most parents experience it at some point during their child's life. Most parents do not recognize it until they have moved past the stage. If someone you respect and trust feels you may be in denial, receive professional counseling and support so you can move beyond denial and participate better in your child's care. Be understanding if your spouse or other family members are experiencing denial. Help them receive the assistance they need to deal with their feelings.

**Feeling Guilty**
Almost all parents of children with cerebral palsy have felt guilty at certain times in their child's life. Most parents have a secret fear that something they did must have caused their child's serious disability. Some parents or grandparents may feel that a child's disability is a punishment for their own past sins.

Most families need a great deal of reassurance that nothing they did or did not do caused their child's disability. If a parent did engage in a behavior that may have contributed to their child's disability, such as heavy drinking or taking drugs during pregnancy, it is important for the parent to receive the help needed to lead a safer, healthier life. This helps the parent give the baby all the help and support it will require.

**Feeling Cheated**
Most parents are surprised to find they feel somehow cheated. They expected to have a perfectly normal baby who would do many things that now may never come to pass. Before the baby is born, parents carry a fantasy baby in their minds and hearts that is perfect in every way. The fantasy baby is often intellectually gifted, a famous athlete, a beautiful bride, or a successful professional. Now, parents must deal with the death and loss of the

perfect fantasy baby. For all families, this is the death of a dream. It is a painful process. Time is needed to love and accept the strengths and weaknesses of the real baby gradually.

**Feeling Anger**

Often when the protection of denial is gone, parents feel very angry. Why did this terrible thing have to happen to our family? Why our child? Parents often quickly look for someone to blame. Did a doctor do something to harm my child? Was I exposed to some chemical where I work? Did I catch a virus or an infection at the grocery store? During these times of angry feelings, parents are sometimes frustrated and bitter. Parents may file lawsuits or lash out at professionals. Try to sort out your emotions, speak, and act very carefully when you feel angry. Often, a parent can feel very angry and not even realize it. Parent support groups can be very helpful at this point, allowing families to express and share their feelings.

**Bargaining**

In an attempt to deal with a difficult situation, families frequently try to bargain with God, with doctors, or with other professionals participating in their child's care. Parents often pray for their child's complete recovery in exchange for being a perfect person afterward. They sometimes try to bargain with teachers or healthcare professionals. The parents hope that if they give a child a certain medicine or surgery or attend every therapy appointment, the professional can guarantee that their child will begin to speak, sit up alone, or walk without a walker. Unfortunately, no professional can promise that a particular child will achieve a particular skill. Professionals can only help each child to achieve her personal best. Progress is often frustratingly slow. When parents are bargaining, the child with cerebral palsy can become their whole world. They obsessively care for their child, refusing to accept help from others. Bargaining parents may temporarily push even their other children or spouses completely out of their lives. This particularly dangerous reaction can contribute to divorce or depression in other family members. Professional counseling is *very* critical in this situation.

## Acceptance

Thankfully, a wonderful period called acceptance comes in most families lives. The family begins to accept their child's limitations, seeing and appreciating the positives and strengths in their child. Despite the severity of a child's disability, families begin to see how this child does contribute positively to the family and to the community. Often, a child with a disability can bring out the very best qualities in a parent, a brother or sister, or even a neighbor. Families come to realize that they would be incomplete without this very special little person no matter how complicated her care may be. Having a child with cerebral palsy, even with all of the struggles, can shape you into an exceptional parent and a much more sensitive, strong, and productive person.

Families come to see how this special child focuses and enhances the quality of their lives. Parents of children with cerebral palsy do not have time for unimportant things. In time, these families know that professionals can help a child to do her best but cannot cure cerebral palsy. Eventually, families achieve a balance between the child's special needs and the needs and goals of the rest of the family. All family members and frequently friends, neighbors, and professionals participate together in this child's care. Parents learn how to find, train, and allow others to help.

Once acceptance is achieved, families may not stay in that frame of mind forever. Sometimes, a family milestone event such as the year your child would have started kindergarten or a similar-age cousin starts to walk, talk, or drive can retrigger grieving or other stages of adjustment. Just be patient with each other. Keep looking for and using counseling, support, and help in the care of your child.

# 7

# RELATING TO FAMILY, FRIENDS, AND STRANGERS

Relating to family, friends, and strangers can be confusing when you have a child with cerebral palsy. People know exactly how to behave when a family has a normal, healthy baby. They are often awkward, uncertain, and sometimes cruel when a child has a disability.

When dealing with family members, it is important to recognize and support the different patterns of grieving in each person. Encourage family members to talk and seek support from each other, friends, parent support groups, or individual counselors. Realize that feelings of grief may cause a family member to withdraw from the baby or try to take over the baby completely.

At this difficult time, parents are under extreme stress. Parents can react with anger, withdrawal, or denial. It is common to feel very angry or frustrated with your spouse. The additional stress can reek havoc on a strong relationship and can cause a weaker one to collapse. The stress of raising a child with disabilities can also trigger or worsen problems with depression or use of alcohol or drugs. Professionals should be sought immediately to deal with these serious but common problems. Refer to the Keys titled "You and Your Spouse" and "Counseling and Professional Support" for more information. Siblings and grandparents often have a difficult time adjusting to the stress of having a family member with cerebral palsy. Refer to the Keys titled "Brothers and Sisters" and "Grandparents" for many practical suggestions to help them.

Friends, as well as family members, often feel awkward and uncomfortable when a family is going through a difficult change. Many friends will withdraw. They do not know how to help, feel overwhelmed by your child's condition, or feel they will be in the way. Tell your friends that you miss them. Provide information about your child's condition. Educate when you can. Let your friends gradually learn the special needs of your child. Show them something your child really enjoys, such as being rocked, listening to music, playing with a special toy, or looking in a mirror. If your friends want to help, accept their offers. They can be especially helpful with familiar tasks such as picking up your other children from school, baking a casserole, or running errands.

Many friends feel much more comfortable when they feel they are making a useful contribution. Always thank them with a hug or a note expressing how much you appreciate their gesture. If a friend offers to baby-sit your child with cerebral palsy, you are blessed. Make sure you adequately train your friend to provide any special care your child requires.

Dealing with strangers can be a new and challenging experience for a family with a child with cerebral palsy. Expect a certain amount of staring. People frequently stare unintentionally at anything or anyone that is unusual or unexpected. Break the ice by introducing yourself and your child. Make a positive comment with your greeting. For example, "Johnny is really enjoying his ride in his wheelchair today. He listened to the birds in the park." If a stranger asks an unwelcome question, try to answer positively and accurately. Keep your answer short and simple, then move on. Humor can be very helpful in dealing with uncomfortable questions. If a stranger showers pity on you or your child, thank him for his concern, but always point out at least one of your child's strengths or accomplishments. Never let your child hear himself called a burden by anyone, even if your child cannot speak.

## RELATING TO FAMILY, FRIENDS, AND STRANGERS

As soon as you possibly can, teach your child about his disability. Role-play with him about how to introduce himself and explain his disability to other children and adults. A simple but accurate and quick explanation can make it much easier for a child to make new friends and be accepted. An example of a simple explanation is, "I was born very early, and my brain got hurt, and it makes it hard for me to walk."

Remember that today's strangers may be tomorrow's friends and helpers. Many successful medical professionals are led to the field by an ill or disabled family member or friend that they met during childhood. As much as possible, bring your child with you to school, to church, and into the community. Together you educate, inform, and enlighten the world just by being there.

# 8

# GETTING TO KNOW OTHER PARENTS

When you find out that your child has cerebral palsy, you may feel as if your child is the only one in the world with it. That is definitely not the case. Among children who are disabled, cerebral palsy is a common diagnosis. It is comforting to meet other families on a similar journey. The community has many places where you are likely to meet parents of other children with cerebral palsy.

A children's hospital is such a place. The neurology, orthopedic, physical therapy, or occupational therapy departments may care for many children with cerebral palsy. The social workers in a children's hospital may be able to help you locate parent support groups in your area.

Community rehabilitation centers, especially those that specialize in working with children, are excellent resources for finding many families. The United Cerebral Palsy Association, the Easter Seal Society, or the March of Dimes frequently provide services to children with cerebral palsy out of community-based rehabilitation centers.

The special education department of your local school district often serves many children with cerebral palsy. These children frequently receive special education services; educational testing; physical, occupational, and speech therapy; and special services for vision and hearing problems. Parents can often form their own formal or informal groups as their children share classrooms, therapy, or Special Olympics together.

Early intervention programs provide an excellent opportunity to meet other parents of children with developmental delays like cerebral palsy. A variety of organizations serve families of children with cerebral palsy. State Rehabilitation Commissions frequently serve adults and some children with cerebral palsy. Programs for people with mental retardation serve some adults and children with cerebral palsy. They frequently have family support programs such as respite care or caregiver support groups. Your state, city, or local Department of Health and Human Services may be able to provide a listing of programs in your area for families dealing with cerebral palsy. Your child's doctor, the hospital emergency room, or the medical clinic your child attends may be able to help you find appropriate support groups or link you with other families they serve.

The public library can be a great place to find information about locating other families with similar circumstances. A computer search of the topics *cerebral palsy* and *parent support* should provide lists of published information.

The National Information Center for Children and Youth with Disabilities (NICHCY) provides parent support group information. It can be reached by toll-free telephone, voice/teletype, or Internet. *Exceptional Parent Magazine* is also available in larger public or medical libraries and by subscription. It provides parents of children with disabilities information about products, services, programs, and parent support.

Parents of children with cerebral palsy can participate in larger formal support groups. The Mother's United for Moral Support (MUMS), the National Father's Network, and the Sibling Support Project provide newsletters and information.

With a little determination, your family can reach out and meet other families in your community who share the bond of having a child with cerebral palsy. The friendships formed can be some of the most treasured relationships in life. Many of the resources mentioned here are listed in the resource section of this book. You can receive information about local chapters by contacting these national organizations.

# 9

# COUNSELING AND PROFESSIONAL SUPPORT

Finding out that a child has cerebral palsy can be a very stressful time in a family's life. Often, it is very healthy and necessary for one or several family members to meet with a professional counselor to sort out painful feelings or problems with how the family functions. If a family is already stressed with several other children, single parenthood, divorce, an unhappy marriage, unemployment, financial problems, an ill or aged family member, drug or alcohol problems, mental illness, depression, or a difficult teenager in the home, the added stress of having a child with cerebral palsy can be enough to blow a family apart. Divorce rates are high among couples raising a child with a disability. For these reasons, a family should not hesitate to use professional support services.

Professional counseling support can come in many forms. Professional counselors, social workers, marriage or family counselors or therapists, ministers, psychologists, and psychiatrists can play important roles in helping family members adjust and redesign their lives in times of stress. Whenever you are considering consulting a mental health professional, ask when and where the professional was trained and what special licenses, degrees, or certifications that professional holds. Ask what professional organizations the person belongs to. Find out how much experience he has working with families who have children with disabilities. Always call or write to make certain the therapist or counselor has indeed received the credentials he claims. Ask to speak with other families who have met with the counselor. Were they satisfied? Did the professional help the family map out concrete actions to help the family cope? Were they taught how to handle conflict and stress or how to fight fairly? Did the counselor help them locate resources? Often, a program that works with your child, your child's doctor, or your family's physician can refer a professional counselor.

Always check your family's health insurance benefits to see what, if any, professional mental health and counseling benefits are available. Some children's rehabilitation or hospital programs offer counseling at low or no cost. Always make sure charges for counseling are clear and in writing before services begin.

Many times, the love and support of family, friends, church members, and a good parent support group can provide the warmth and support that your family needs in order to thrive. In times of crisis, families of children with cerebral palsy should not fail to ask for the professional, compassionate support they need.

# PART THREE

# BALANCING FAMILY RELATIONSHIPS

Part Three addresses the whole family. It encourages parents to make time for each other and share the responsibilities of parenting a child with cerebral palsy. Part Three shows how to make siblings feel special, too. The decision whether or not to add another child to the family is discussed as are issues pertaining to single parents. You will learn how using day care and respite care can help you to balance your time and family. This part contains a special Key about the role grandparents play in supporting parents and nurturing special grandchildren.

# 10

# EVERYONE IN YOUR FAMILY IS SPECIAL

One very important job of parents is to help build their child's feelings of self-worth. Every child must feel special and valuable in order to grow up healthy and well adjusted. A few tips can help parents of children with cerebral palsy accomplish this most important task.

Look for positives in your child's development. Talk with other family members about what is wonderful about your child. No quality is too small or too unimportant to mention. Does your child have a sweet smile? Does she make happy, squealing noises when you enter a room? Does she love to be held and rocked? Does she love to have a bath? Did your child just master scooting around on the floor? Does she try hard to stand when you hold her hands?

Give encouragement, hugs, and lots of love to reward good behavior and accomplishments. All of your children, whether they have disabilities or not, need to know that you are proud of them for what they have done and what they have tried to do.

Avoid talking negatively in front of your child. Always assume that your child can understand what you say, even if she cannot speak. Children with cerebral palsy are often very sensitive to nonverbal communication or body language. They often stiffen or cry because of angry voices or sudden, abrupt handling. They can tell when you or others around them are angry, resentful, or upset. Never discuss your frustrations, anger, or disappointment about your child's condition in the presence of your child, assuming that she does not understand what you are saying. Do not allow other people to say negative things about your child in her presence, either. Instead of saying your child *cannot* do something, say your child can do something with a certain type of help or equipment. Do not use painful words like helpless, burden, retard, vegetable, crippled, dumb, or stupid to describe your child.

Sometimes, people wish to express their sympathy for the difficulties your child and family are facing. They can smother you and your child with words of pity. A typical comment is, "Oh, poor little Jenny. It's so tragic. I just don't know how you can take it." The best way to respond is with a positive statement about your child's most recent accomplishment. For example say, "Thanks for your concern, but we are so happy and proud. Jenny is learning to sit up by herself." When your child overhears your positive statement about her progress, she learns that you are as proud of her as she is of her accomplishments. This builds her self-confidence.

Celebrating small accomplishments can help a child with cerebral palsy feel very special. Bake a cake together to celebrate your child's first day at a special school. Make a card or banner when your child graduates from bottle to trainer cup or from walker to crutches. Reward your child with stickers or, occasionally, with an inexpensive toy such as bubbles or chunky crayons for a job well done. Take pictures and display them when your child first learns how to activate a switch toy or use a computer.

Your family should celebrate signs of improved health such as a week without seizures, no longer needing the apnea monitor, breathing without a ventilator, feeding without a tube, or gaining weight. Celebrations can be as elaborate as a party or as small as a hug, a special cookie, or noting an accomplishment on a calendar.

Include your child in all special occasions such as birthdays, holidays, and family events. If your child cannot take part because of illness or length of travel, let her participate by making a small gift for the occasion. Bring a picture or a letter describing your special child's recent accomplishments, school, or new friends to share with others. Whenever the rest of your family dresses up to celebrate, dress up your child with cerebral palsy. A new outfit, a different hairstyle, hairbows, or a shiny new pair of shoes can make a child with cerebral palsy feel beautiful or handsome. You can also decorate special equipment such as braces, wheelchairs, or oxygen tanks.

Another important part of making your child feel special is to respect your child's developing personality. Many commonly believe that children with disabilities do not have individual personalities and preferences about what is going on around them. Do not assume that your child does not care what she does, where she goes, or who she goes with. If your child smiles and laughs when she is swung, take her to the park or build a special backyard swing. If your child loves the water, host her birthday party at the pool and let her splash along with the other children while wearing a life preserver and cool sunglasses. If your child likes the color red, make sure her new wheelchair and crutches are red, even if mom and dad prefer blue. Encourage your child to choose music, toys, food, activities, positions, TV shows, and entertainment. Your child may express her choice through eye gaze, a sound that means yes or no, touching a desired object, or by simply becoming excited when something happens that she likes. Encouraging all those methods of communication and respecting your child's interests will make her feel special.

In addition to your child with special needs, every other family member needs to feel special. By using friends, relatives, respite care, or a hired baby-sitter, make a point of spending individual time with each of your immediate family members at least once a month. Husbands and wives also need special time alone together to nurture their relationship. Each child needs separate time alone with mom and with dad in order to grow up feeling special. Special time does not have to be elaborate or expensive. It can be as a simple as a long walk together or an ice cream cone in the park. During special time, the parent must be completely available to the child, without the demands of home, job, or other family members. This is very important for siblings and will be discussed in Key 12.

Bringing your child with cerebral palsy into the world of school, work, church, and neighborhood along with your other children shows that she is also a vital, important part of your family. Just being included like other children is a simple yet important way a parent can make any child feel special.

# 11

# YOU AND YOUR SPOUSE

When a couple gives birth to or adopts a healthy child, the couple's relationship permanently changes. Parenthood brings joys and challenges that the couple has never dealt with before. The new parents learn to manage crying, disrupted sleep, feeding schedules, piles of diapers and laundry, hiring babysitters, finding a good day care center, returning to school or work, temper tantrums, childproofing their home, and doctor visits for minor illnesses.

When a couple gives birth to or adopts a child with cerebral palsy, the couple may face all of those issues plus a great deal more. Instead of occasional doctor visits for colds or shots, the child may require extensive hospital stays or long-term therapy. Medical costs may be very high. Large amounts of time may be devoted to taking your child to see various medical specialists. Your life may seem like an endless list of appointments.

You may feel like your home has been invaded. Some children with cerebral palsy need nearly constant supervision because of medical complications. You may feel as if you have no privacy as a couple if you now share your home with home health nurses and therapists. Instead of a nursery with a simple crib and toys, you may be stepping over IV poles, feeding pumps, apnea monitors, a ventilator, a suction machine, a stander, a walker, a wheelchair, and braces.

All of these sudden and unexpected changes can place a great deal of stress on parents and can severely damage a relationship. Divorce rates are higher than average in families with children who are disabled. Special attention to the marriage is required to protect it from the strains of raising a child with special needs.

You and your spouse may face a lot of fear. You wonder how serious your child's disability will be. Will your child be able to walk, talk, or care for himself? Will your child be able to live away from home? The fear and uncertainty you face can cause you and your partner to feel overwhelmed, short-tempered, depressed, and angry.

Many parents handle their grief differently, further stressing the marriage. One parent may cope with the stress by becoming very busy with all of the child's care. The other parent may avoid the child or, perhaps, avoid being at home by working long hours or spending time with friends or hobbies. If you understand that these are all normal reactions to a very stressful situation, it is easier to be patient with your partner. Parents should also encourage their spouse to receive all the help needed to cope with the situation. This may include counseling.

Provided that you are in a healthy, loving relationship, one of the most important ways you can show love to your special child is to show you love his other parent. All children thrive when they live in a home with two loving parents who can handle a challenging situation well together. Sometimes, it is helpful for each parent to write a list of what things they could do to make this situation easier. Some items on your lists might be

- Find someone to baby-sit one night a week.
- Try to schedule all medical appointments on one particular day.
- Get away for a weekend together at least every three months.
- Find other parents going through similar situations.
- Meet some families of adults with cerebral palsy so you can better know what to expect when your child grows older.
- Take turns with duties like housekeeping, mowing the lawn, and staying home when your child is ill.

You can easily become so caught up in the needs of your child with cerebral palsy that you ignore your partner and marriage. If you are in a healthy, loving relationship, keeping that relationship strong and happy is one of the most important supports you can provide your child.

If you are in an unhealthy relationship, such as an abusive or violent marriage, or in a home with stressors, such as alcohol abuse, or drug abuse, or mental illness, those problems should be addressed immediately with the help of a professional. Never be afraid to ask for help. Your child's doctor, hospital social worker, case manager, or therapists may be able to help you find the assistance you and your family need and deserve. Refer to Key 9 for more information on counseling and professional support.

In the beginning, it can be painful and difficult for you and your partner to learn that your child has a disability. As time goes on, however, many parents find that their marriage and their lives were greatly enriched by overcoming the challenges together, with their child.

# 12

# BROTHERS AND SISTERS

Brothers and sisters of children with cerebral palsy may react strongly to having a sibling with a disability in their home. Brothers and sisters may have different emotional reactions at different stages of their lives. This depends somewhat on whether they are the eldest, youngest, or one of many siblings.

In the beginning, brothers and sisters may have the same response as any child to a new baby. Toddlers tend to act less mature by showing more babylike behaviors when the new baby arrives. Temper tantrums, bedwetting, thumb sucking, or whining may appear as a sibling has to compete for mom's or dad's attention.

When a baby has cerebral palsy, however, the demands on a parent's time can be enormous and will last much longer, possibly a lifetime. When a parent's attention is greatly focused on a baby with special needs, a brother or sister will usually feel pushed aside at least temporarily. A sibling may spend more time cared for by school, day care, friends, or relatives while the family meets the unexpected needs of the child with cerebral palsy. As a result, the sibling may feel ignored, forgotten, or angry.

Some brothers and sisters respond to this stress by becoming very quiet and withdrawn. Some respond by becoming angry, babyish, demanding, or by clinging to the parents. All of these responses are fairly normal; however, parents should be very sensitive to and aware of the emotional needs of their children who are not disabled. At any age, brothers and sisters may need special support and counseling, too. Sibling support groups are becoming popular across the country.

Expect that your other children, both younger and older, will resent the large amount of time and attention your child with cerebral palsy receives. Regularly use baby-sitters or respite care to allow you some individual time with each of your other children. Do not cancel your dates with them. Spending quality time alone with each child will send the message that all of your children are important and special.

Eventually, a brother or sister will try to bond with the child who has cerebral palsy. Give them a chance to play together or just simply be together and touch one another while you watch from a distance. Do not criticize the brother's or sister's attempt to play with the baby. Many just give up if scolded or told they are too rough. Try to show them ways to enjoy toys or music together. Praise your children's efforts. Also, give simple and truthful explanations for all the questions that your children ask about their sibling with cerebral palsy.

Find simple ways for brothers and sisters to help care for their sibling. They can help choose toys, clothes, room decorations, and colors of medical equipment. They can bring things like diapers or braces to their parents when needed. However, you also need to encourage your children to allow their special sibling to do things by herself and make her own choices, even if it takes extra time or the child with cerebral palsy seems slow or clumsy. Sometimes, brothers and sisters can help too much, which keeps their sibling from practicing new and difficult skills.

Do not expect your nondisabled children to be quiet, good, and perfectly behaved at all times just because you have a child with cerebral palsy who makes extra demands on you. Under these circumstances, it is common for stressed parents to be short-tempered or to expect too much from the children who do not have a disability. Do not turn siblings into substitute parents by giving them inappropriate adult responsibilities. Examples include having a sibling feed a child who has difficulty eating or give medications, or asking

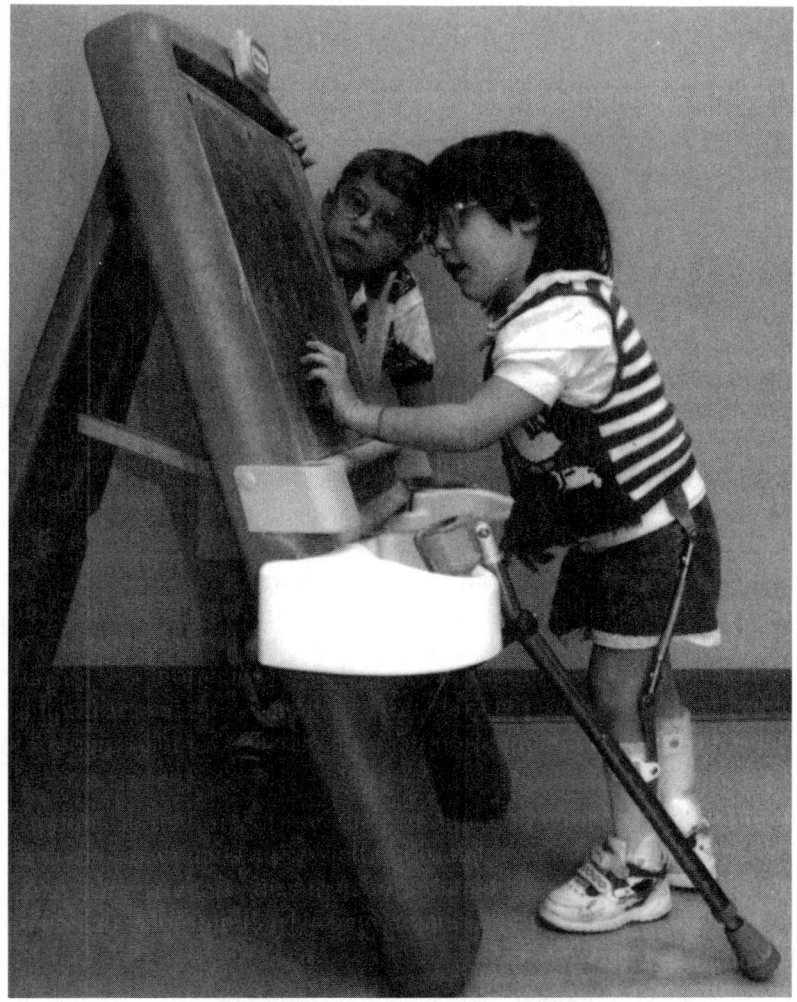

**I like to play with my brother.**

a brother or sister to baby-sit when the child's care is complex. Take your children's age and maturity into consideration before allowing them to take care of their sibling. Older children can help with a sibling who is disabled but should not be responsible for a great deal of caregiving. They need a chance to be children, too.

Be consistent in how you discipline and reward your children. Do not allow verbal or physical abuse between siblings regardless of disability. The child with cerebral palsy should not be allowed to hit or otherwise hurt another sibling. Time-out, discipline, or rewards like sticker charts can be useful for *all* your children.

The school years can be especially difficult for siblings of a person with cerebral palsy. At this time, children are noticing differences in each other and their classmates' families. They are easily affected by teasing. Do not force your nondisabled children to play with their sibling when friends visit. Allow them to make that choice on their own. Often, brothers and sisters will build a special but sometimes private relationship when given the chance to be together after friends have gone home.

Older children, especially preteens and teenagers, can be very embarrassed by having a brother or sister who is different. This is a normal stage of adolescent development. They may feel unable to cope with possible questions from and teasing by their peers that encountering their sibling with cerebral palsy might bring. Provide information, when appropriate, that will make your adolescent children and their friends feel more comfortable. Let them choose whether or not to involve the sibling in their activities. You might be surprised to find your children hanging out at the mall or renting movies together.

Do not burden or frighten your nondisabled children by saying that they may have to care for your child with cerebral palsy if something happens to you. Children should never have to fear an overwhelming adult responsibility. When planning for the future care of your child with cerebral palsy, you should investigate and plan for several options. Only an adult brother or sister can decide to care for a sibling with cerebral palsy. This should be only one of several possible choices.

Having twins, triplets, and larger multiple births adds an extraordinary challenge to parenting. Cerebral palsy makes things even more complicated. Sometimes, one twin or triplet will have cerebral palsy. Other times, both or all three will be affected. Their conditions and abilities may be similar or one child may be more involved than the others.

Because children born at the same time, like twins and triplets, usually have a strong bond between them, you may not have to help them build a relationship as you do with other siblings. However, your children may need support in other ways. A healthy twin may feel guilty or neglected. A twin who is more involved than the other may wonder, "Why me?" Parents may expect more from a child with mild cerebral palsy than they do from a twin who is more disabled. They may give the child with more extensive needs more attention and assume that the other twin is doing fine because she can do more by herself. However, this child or young adult may actually need more emotional support for dealing with her disability, going to school, and thinking about the future.

Parents should make sure that they pay attention to the needs of all of their children and not become completely absorbed by the needs of a child with cerebral palsy. Resist the temptation to compare any of your children. Each child is unique and has her own special needs regardless of disability. Take special care to spend time as a family to celebrate the accomplishments of each brother and sister. Through encouragement and an understanding of their similarities and differences, you can help your children bond and form a lasting relationship.

## 13

# GRANDPARENTS

Many people do not realize how upsetting it may be for a grandparent to have a grandchild with cerebral palsy. For some grandparents, the pain, fear, and grief may be nearly as intense as the parents'. Some grandparents respond by avoiding the grandchild with cerebral palsy. Some grandparents deny that anything is wrong with the child. A few grandparents turn their anger onto the child's parents. Grandparents may believe that a behavior of one or both parents caused the child's disability. The stress of having a child with a disability join the family can cause old hurts and conflicts to surface.

A common reaction for some grandparents is to "take over the baby." This is a typical reaction of a grieving grandparent with a firstborn grandchild, especially if the parents are young or inexperienced. Grandparents are often so eager to help in such a difficult time that they may unintentionally cause parents to feel incapable of taking care of the child or to feel disconnected from the child.

Grandparents can constructively do many things to help. The most important thing is to reassure and emotionally support the baby's parents. Put aside any family quarrels as best you can. Some families find it useful to have a family meeting. Grandparents should ask the child's parents what they can *specifically* do to help.

Grandparents can help in many ways. They can gather information about cerebral palsy or available treatment programs. Grandparents can provide transportation or emotional support for doctor and therapy appointments. They can sometimes help with a family's financial needs. They can provide child care or activities for brothers and sisters. Grandparents can care for the child with cerebral palsy if a parent needs to return to work or needs a break. Supporting both of the baby's parents and their marriage is perhaps the most important thing grandparents can do.

Another critical job for grandparents is to build a relationship with the grandchild. The love, attention, and companionship grandparents can provide can cause a child with cerebral palsy to bloom. No matter how great the child's disabilities, as a grandparent, you can always connect by rocking a child in a rocking chair or pushing a child in a stroller to the park. Learn as much as possible about your grandchild's daily care routine so you will feel comfortable helping with feeding, carrying, bathing, or giving medication. Take your time getting to know your grandchild. Do not feel rushed. Relax and enjoy this precious little one. Read books and magazines to find out more about cerebral palsy. Attend therapy when you can to cheer on your grandchild. Meet other families who have children with cerebral palsy. Befriend another grandparent of a child with cerebral palsy. You may have a lot in common.

# 14

# RESPITE CARE AND DAY CARE

No matter how much you love your children or how much they need you, like all parents you need to take a break now and then. Some parents have a break from their children when they go to work or when the children are in school, but, often, this is not enough. Some parents of children with disabilities do not even have those short times away from their responsibilities.

**Respite Care**

Having free time to do necessary and enjoyable activities is important for mental health. Parents also need to spend time with their spouse or significant other without dealing with the responsibilities of children. Additionally, siblings of children with disabilities need time alone with their parents where they can also feel special. Some parents may have other family members or friends who will supervise the children. Often, however, parents feel that it would be a burden to ask family or friends for help. Parents may feel that no one else has the training needed to care for a child with cerebral palsy. For these reasons and many others, families often turn to respite care.

The word *respite* literally means temporary relief. In this book, *respite* and *respite care* identify services available to families or primary care providers of people with disabilities. Respite care services are provided through a variety of resources or agencies depending on the state in which you live. Speak with your child's case manager or social worker about resources in your community. You may also want to contact your local Department of Health and Human Services or State Developmental Disabilities Council for information. Churches and schools may also provide these services. Costs depend on the organization. Other resources can be found at the back of this book.

Respite care is a temporary or short-term way for parents or care providers to take some time off from caring for a person with a disability. Federal laws passed in 1988 and 1989, the *Children's Justice Act* and the *Children with Disability Temporary Care Reauthorization Act,* support respite care. Although these laws provide financial assistance to states for respite care programs, the resources are limited. Depending on the provider agency, you may have to qualify for services. The amount of respite time varies depending on your individual needs. You can request respite care for a few hours at a time to attend appointments, spend an evening with your spouse, and so on. You can also request respite care for longer time periods for activities like a vacation. Respite care is also available in the case of family emergencies.

A respite care provider has training much like a home health aide who cares for elderly or ill people. Interview the provider to make sure that he or she has the specific skills necessary to care for your child's special needs. Ask the organization for references and procedures for dealing with emergencies. Make sure that you and your child are comfortable with the provider, and that the provider is comfortable in your home and knows where things are kept. Spend time together before leaving your child and the provider alone. Use a similar approach to see if out-of-home respite care is appropriate for your child. Lastly, do not feel guilty about needing and using respite care. By taking time off, you will have more energy to be a better parent.

**Day Care**

Day care for your child may be a necessity because you work. It may be a luxury because you need time to yourself or want your child to spend time with other children. Unfortunately, finding day care for children with cerebral palsy can be very difficult.

Obviously, family, friends, a nanny, or respite care can babysit your child. If you are interested in day care or a child care facility, your best bet may be talking with other parents of children with cerebral palsy. Your phone book's listings for child care may not identify facilities that take children with disabilities. Although legally through the *Americans with Disabilities Act* a facility that accepts federal government funds cannot discriminate against your child because of disability, the staff may not be trained to work with children who have disabilities. You can call and receive information from various facilities or use a child care referral source in your community. Check with local churches and civic organizations to see what is available. Easter Seals centers often offer day care for children with and without disabilities.

After determining your options, visit the day care centers and check them with the Better Business Bureau. Decide if you want your child to be only with others who have disabilities or also with children who are developing normally. Being with children who do not have disabilities can be motivating and educational for all of the children.

Check the day care facility's activities, curriculum, and staff-to-child ratio. Each staff member should supervise a low number of children, preferably no more than three or four. The number may need to be lower if several children in the group have disabilities.

You should insist that your day care location be inspected for safety, be childproofed, and only have staff who are currently certified in infant and child cardiopulmonary resuscitation (CPR). Your day care provider should be fully trained by you or members of your child's treatment team to feed, dress, play with, position, toilet, and medicate your child in the most safe and therapeutic way possible. The provider should also be trained to operate any special equipment.

Finding appropriate day care can be a time-consuming process for any parent. Take the time to provide your child with a safe and stimulating environment. It will be well worth the effort.

# 15

# SHOULD WE HAVE ANOTHER BABY?

The decision to have any child is personal, made between a loving couple, and should always be considered carefully and thoughtfully. The decision can be made more confusing and complex when the family already includes a child with a disability.

A key question to ask yourself is, "Did we want another child before our child with cerebral palsy was born?" Parents of a child with cerebral palsy should be careful not to fall into a common trap. Many parents, as part of their grieving process, feel a strong urge to give birth to a perfect, nondisabled child. This drive to produce a perfect, healthy baby can be strong and difficult to ignore. As a normal part of grief, parents can impulsively create another baby in an attempt to test their bodies and prove that they are capable of producing a normal child. This "replacement" child further stresses the family. The family has the added responsibilities of caring for another infant when it has not resolved the pain and grief felt facing the challenge of raising the child with cerebral palsy.

Parents can subconsciously be driven to have more children by their fear of no one caring for their child with special needs when they can no longer do so. Siblings cannot be forced to care for their brother or sister with cerebral palsy. Living with a sibling is only one of many possible living arrangements. Having another child as an insurance plan to care for a brother or sister with cerebral palsy is placing an unfair burden on the nondisabled child. Each child deserves to be wanted for her own unique purpose in life.

When making the sensitive decision of whether or not to have another child, a couple should always make informed decisions. Cerebral palsy itself is not an inherited condition; however, many children have movement and development disorders that may be mislabeled as cerebral palsy that are indeed genetic disorders and can be inherited by additional children. Parents should be certain whether or not their child's motor and development problems are caused by an inherited or genetic problem before future pregnancies occur. Your child's physician can be very helpful in providing this information or arranging for genetic counseling or testing, if necessary. Never hesitate to receive a second medical opinion if you still feel uncertain.

Anytime a family considers having another child, a careful review of the whole family system is appropriate. Does the family have adequate time, money, and resources to devote a lifetime of caring to another child? Is the family under stress? Is the marriage strong and healthy? Are there sufficient financial resources to raise another child? Do both parents agree that they want another child at this time? The very best reason to have another child is that after careful thought and planning, a family is ready to face all the joys and challenges that an additional child will add to your special and precious family.

# 16

# SINGLE-PARENT FAMILY CONCERNS

Any parent of a child with cerebral palsy can feel stressed and tired by the many challenges a parent faces. A single parent, however, can feel even more overwhelmed. A two-parent family can more easily divide the load. A single parent has to develop a strong support system in order to best meet the needs of the child and family.

A common problem faced by most single parents is the need to work outside the home in addition to providing twenty-four hour a day supervision to a child with special needs. It is impossible for any one person to work outside the home and provide around-the-clock care, so other solutions must be found.

Many single parents report their greatest problem is finding reliable day care that will accept a child with disabilities. Many parents are unaware that children with cerebral palsy will qualify to attend early childhood intervention programs at their local public school. Center-based intervention is typically available to children once they are two or three years old. Early childhood programs are available at the local school district level from birth for children with vision and hearing problems in addition to their cerebral palsy. Many of these programs are not necessarily full-day or five-day-per-week programs.

Your state's Department of Health also maintains a list of registered day homes and licensed day care centers, which are grouped by county or zip code. Some day care centers and many private registered day homes will accept a child with cerebral palsy after discussing the child's needs in detail with the parent and meeting the child personally. They must also obtain any necessary training for meeting the child's special needs.

Other problems for single parents include: What am I going to do if a family emergency occurs? How am I ever going to go on a date, enjoy a weekend away from home, or take a vacation? Respite care is absolutely necessary for a single-parent family with a child who is disabled. Key 14 contains information about respite care.

Another single-parent concern is how to cope with the physical demands of lifting and carrying a child with cerebral palsy, especially as the child grows older and heavier. Special adaptive equipment for lifting, bathing, transporting, and positioning can be very helpful. Consult with your child's physician and therapists. The best way to protect your child's ability to live at home successfully is to protect your mental and physical health and prevent back injuries.

Single parents must often balance the needs of other children in the home. Finding friends and extended family members to help mentor your other children can go a long way toward meeting your children's needs. Maintaining open communication with your children's other parent and side of the family can also provide resources for you. This may be difficult to do, but it is worth the extra effort when the emotional health and welfare of your children are at stake.

When a single parent cares for a child with cerebral palsy, that parent may be secretly afraid that he will never find a partner willing to accept the special needs of his child. Many single parents of children with disabilities do remarry or form warm and loving relationships with new partners. You need to develop a support network that will allow you to go into your community and meet potential partners. Your prospective new partner must see you successfully balancing the needs of your child within the total framework of your life. Caring for a child with cerebral palsy is an important part of your life, but it is not your entire life. Many new partners are attracted and bonded to the parent of a child with special needs by those qualities you possess as a special parent—strength, love, commitment, patience, sacrifice, and caring. These are ideal qualities for a life partner. Do not forget that your child has magical qualities all his own despite his disabilities. Many people will see the specialness of his spirit.

Financial burdens are often heavier for single-parent families. Consult a social worker or case manager as early as possible to investigate the many programs that might provide food, housing, medical care, money, valuable services, or equipment for your child. Consulting a lawyer familiar with estate planning for families with children who are disabled can also be invaluable. Early planning can greatly help a single parent meet the long-term financial needs of a child with cerebral palsy. For a single parent with a child who has cerebral palsy, life can be challenging but very rewarding. Building a community network including family, friends, teachers, professionals, day care providers, church members, and social services can be the key to success.

# PART FOUR

## YOUR CHILD'S TOTAL WELL-BEING

In Part Four, issues relating to health and development are discussed. You will learn how cerebral palsy may affect your child's physical, mental, and social development. Part Four identifies health problems your child may face, as well as how to address these problems through adequate nutrition, therapy, and new medical techniques. It also introduces you to the members of your child's healthcare team.

# 17

# WHAT IS NORMAL DEVELOPMENT?

Normal development describes how and when children typically learn new skills called milestones. Normal development varies greatly. This accounts for the differences within any group of children at a given age. For example, all twelve month olds do not have the same exact skills. Some walk, others crawl, and yet others run.

Through many years of research and clinical studies, a variety of people have written literature on the normal age ranges for development of fine and gross motor skills, cognitive or mental skills, language skills, and much more. This Key highlights a few big milestones between ages zero to thirty-six months in fine and gross motor skills and language. These are guidelines not absolutes. All children vary in their development. Also, in a child with cerebral palsy, development may not only be slower but also sporadic. Other factors such as health and medications may interfere with the progression of development. Further, look at how your child moves or the quality of her movement. Many children with cerebral palsy will attain a milestone, such as rolling or walking, but they do so with abnormal motor or movement patterns. You need to encourage independent movement, but you also need to teach normal movement patterns or normalization of the skill.

**Basics of Normal Development**

Between birth and three months of age, a baby's interaction with the world is noted by her ability to watch a person or objects and react to sounds and voices by turning her head or startling. Language consists mostly of crying. Motor skills are limited to turning the head left or right and random kicking. At approximately three to four months, she will pick her head up when lying on her stomach, play with her hands in the middle of her chest, and begin to coo. By four to five months, she can roll from her stomach to her back, hold an object, and laugh. At six months, an infant usually can roll from back to stomach, move objects from one hand to the other, sit using hands to prop herself, and babble (ba-ba, da-da). Between seven and nine months, crawling will begin. She can now bang two objects together and will shout for attention. Ten to eleven month olds will be pulling to stand, cruising along furniture, waving bye-bye, and letting go of objects on purpose. Walking usually starts anywhere from ten to fifteen months.

By one year, fine motor skills include picking up small objects like Cheerios, pointing, and putting objects into a container. Language development has progressed to using one-word sentences, making sounds to indicate needs, and saying a few words besides ma-ma and da-da. By eighteen months, a child can walk upstairs with one hand held (and downstairs by twenty-one months). She can scribble with a crayon and build a three-block tower. Her vocabulary has increased to ten to twelve words, and she can name at least one body part.

At twenty-four months, a toddler runs fairly well, draws in a circular motion, strings a few beads, and uses two-word sentences. Riding a tricycle, walking upstairs by herself, having basic use of scissors, saying three-word sentences, and having a vocabulary of fifty or more words all describe a child at thirty months. By three years, a child can climb a jungle gym, build a nine-block tower, copy a circle, answer simple questions, and has 200 or more words in her vocabulary.

Table 1 lists the milestones in motor and language development in children zero to thirty-six months of age. Many other areas such as social, emotional, and cognitive skills measure developmental progression. Children with cerebral palsy may attain some developmental milestones within the usual time periods. Others may come when your child is older. Some developmental skills may never be achieved, whereas others can be done with assistance, equipment, or in your child's own unique way.

## Table 1
## DEVELOPMENTAL MILESTONES

| Age in Months | Gross Motor | Fine Motor | Language |
|---|---|---|---|
| 0–3 | turns head when on back | moves both arms at same time | cries in response to hunger and pain |
| 3–6 | holds head up when on stomach | bats at objects | coos and laughs |
| 6–9 | sits independently | bangs two objects together, keeps hands open | babbles to people |
| 9–12 | crawls and pulls to stand | takes objects out of container, lets go of objects | babbles with inflection |
| 12–15 | walks | picks up small objects, scribbles spontaneously | single-word sentences |
| 15–18 | walks upstairs with one hand held | builds three-block tower | uses 10 to 15 words spontaneously |
| 18–24 | walks downstairs with one hand held | builds four-block tower, imitates circular scribbles | uses two-word sentences, names three pictures |
| 24–30 | walks up and down stairs, rides a tricycle | strings beads, imitates a circle | uses three-word sentences, names five pictures |
| 30–36 | hops on one foot, climbs jungle gym and ladder | imitates a cross, snips on line with scissors | 200 plus words, recites nursery rhymes |

Sources: Setsu Furuno, *HELP Charts* (Palo Alto, CA: VORT Corp., 1994).

Gay L. Pinder, *Developmental Sequence and Connections Among Areas of Motor, Oral Motor, Vocalization, and Cognitive Development from Birth through Four Years* (Seattle, WA: Pinder, 1982).

# 18

# YOUR CHILD'S PHYSICAL DEVELOPMENT

Much like other children, children with cerebral palsy grow and develop at individual and variable rates. They grow taller, gain weight, get bumps and bruises, and go through puberty. A child's physical growth depends on a combination of factors including traits inherited from parents, effects of the environment, and nutrition. If your child has trouble eating, he may be thin and undernourished compared with other children. Also, children with cerebral palsy may grow at a slower rate than other children, depending on what area of the brain is damaged. This may cause puberty to occur late for your child. However, some children with cerebral palsy may go through puberty at an earlier age than usual.

Your child's growth and development will depend on how the brain damage has affected his body. A child who has been affected on just one side or mostly in his legs will look different from a child whose whole body is involved. Cerebral palsy makes a significant impact on a child's ability to move and the stiffness or floppiness of his body parts. Cerebral palsy may most noticeably affect the development of your child's motor skills and the growth of his muscles, joints, and bones.

**Motor Skills**

Everyone has a natural range in the stiffness or floppiness of muscle tone. When a car swerves in front of you while you are driving, your muscle tone increases and you become very stiff or tense. If you have a massage, take a warm bath, or listen to relaxing music, your body will loosen as your muscle tone relaxes. Bodies automatically adjust the amount of muscle tone needed for the activity or emotion. However, the muscle tone of a person with cerebral palsy can rise and fall suddenly from one extreme to the other because of effort or emotion. Your child may have great difficulty controlling his movements because of the stiffness or floppiness of his body. This inability to coordinate movement causes delays in gross and fine motor skill development, which were discussed in Key 17.

A child with cerebral palsy may not learn how to move or perform motor skills in the usual manner. His stiffness, floppiness, or uncoordinated movements may make it difficult to reach for and play with toys or to move his legs independent of each other to crawl. Your child may learn how to perform a motor skill but will tend to always do it in the same fashion. Other children who can control their movements better have a wide variety of options available to them for motor skills. They may be able to sit in a dozen different ways, whereas your child with cerebral palsy might sit only with his legs bent under him like a W. Although your child may use w-sitting, ring sitting, and standing crouched to improve his stability, these postures are bad habits and will limit the development of movement skills. Through therapy and practice, your child can learn different motor patterns and expand his movement options. At least to a certain extent, he can also improve his coordination and gain more control of his body.

**Muscles**

Some children with cerebral palsy have muscles that grow more slowly than their bones. This makes the muscles too short. The muscles may not be as elastic or stretch as easily as muscles in a person without cerebral palsy. Additionally, some children with cerebral palsy lack the normal balance between muscles that allows them to work together. Some muscles pull harder than their partner muscles. Shortening, lack of "stretchiness," and imbalance cause tightness in certain muscles. This tightness will limit movement and result in an inability to bend or straighten a body part completely. These limitations are called *contractures*. The ankle, knee, hip, and elbow joints are the areas most likely to develop contractures in people with cerebral palsy.

## Joints

In addition to contractures, some children with cerebral palsy have other problems with their joints. For example, your child may have hip problems if the thigh bone does not stay in the hip socket. This partial *subluxation* or complete *dislocation* can be very painful and may affect the way your child sits or moves. On the other hand, having a bone "out of joint" may not be painful for your child and may not prevent him from sitting or even from walking. Hip dislocations are common with cerebral palsy. Shoulder and wrist dislocations occur but less often. For various reasons, a person with cerebral palsy may develop joint pain over time. You may need to consider arthritis as a source of pain in the future if your child can no longer do things as well as when he was younger.

## Bones

If a child's muscles pull too hard, his joints are out of place, and he moves in an unusual manner, his bones may not develop normally. Bones may become permanently crooked or twisted. Gravity and poor body position can contribute to deformity.

Some children with cerebral palsy develop a curved spine. A rounded upper back is called *kyphosis*. An *S*- or *C*-shaped curve of the spine is called *scoliosis*. This curvature may be very mild or so severe that the child finds sitting or breathing difficult. Like the spine, feet and hands sometimes become misshapen.

Children with cerebral palsy who are not able to walk are at risk of developing bones that are not as strong as they should be. Activities such as standing and walking that allow your child to hold up his own weight make the bones stronger. Without bearing weight through the bones and moving actively, bones tend to develop osteoporosis. These brittle, fragile bones can break easily.

## Prevention

Some children with cerebral palsy will grow up with only mild physical problems. Others might develop any combination of

## YOUR CHILD'S PHYSICAL DEVELOPMENT

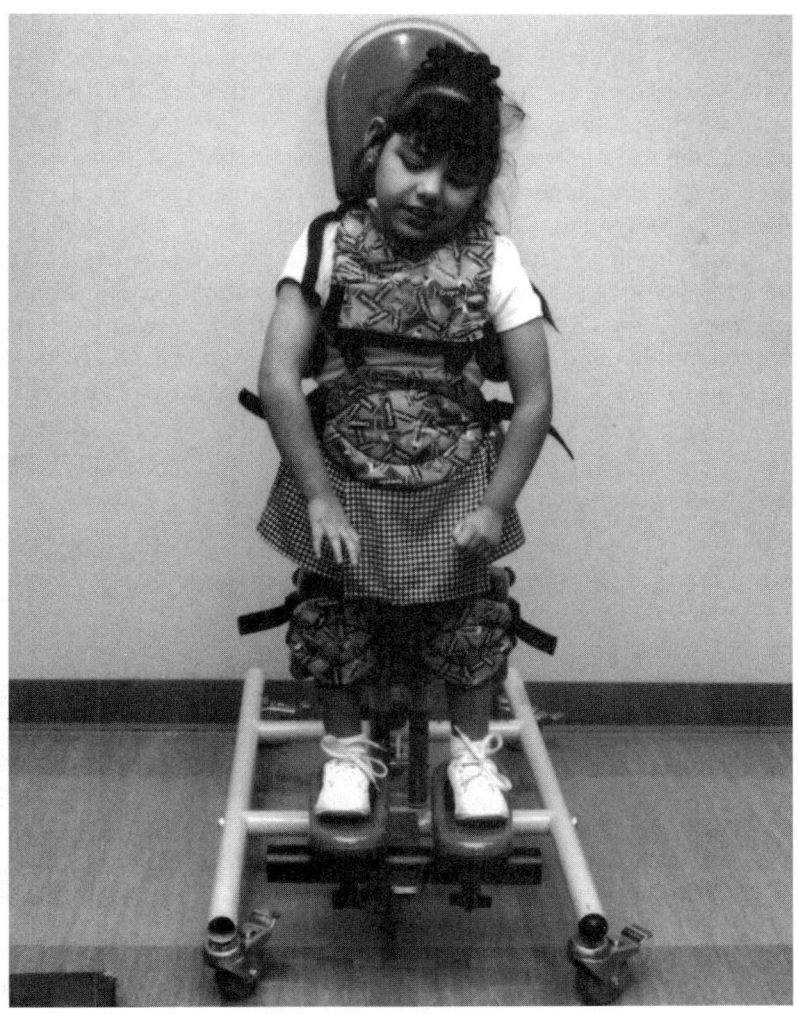

**Practicing standing**

abnormalities of their muscles, joints, and bones. Your child's physician and therapists will help you decide what approach to take to reduce your child's risk of developing the complications discussed in this Key.

An orthopedist may need to see your child regularly to prevent these complications. This doctor will discuss various options with you, which might include therapy, positioning, bracing or splinting, and surgery. Common orthopedic surgeries include spinal stabilization with metal rods to treat scoliosis, *osteotomy* to correct bone alignment or dislocation, and soft tissue release or *tenotomy* to treat contractures. A neurologist may also recommend options for reducing the amount of stiffness or tone your child may have. Key 26 discusses treatments for spasticity. Positioning suggestions are provided in the appendix. Often, a combination of approaches is the most effective way to help a child with cerebral palsy grow and develop without preventable physical problems.

# 19

# YOUR CHILD'S MENTAL DEVELOPMENT

Every parent wonders and worries about how smart their child will be. We all look for those telltale signs to provide clues. Does she make good eye contact? Smile? Play peekaoo? No parent can tell during early infancy how intelligent a child will be. The same holds true for a child diagnosed with cerebral palsy.

Although many people assume that a person with cerebral palsy is always mentally retarded, this is far from the truth. Many people with cerebral palsy, approximately 25 percent, have an average or above average intelligence. *Mental retardation* is a term for significantly low intelligence. It is associated with a person's ability to perform life skills like self-care, communication, safety, self-direction, academics, and work. The degree of severity of mental retardation is based on IQ scores. The four levels of mental retardation are *mild, moderate, severe,* and *profound.* A person with a *learning disability* will have an IQ score within the average to above average range, but test results will show difficulties in specific areas. Learning disabilities interfere with a person's progress in school and in activities of daily living that require reading, writing, and math skills. Fifty to 75 percent of children with cerebral palsy are diagnosed with mental retardation or a learning disability.

In general, mental development emerges or proceeds in a predictable sequence. Professionals often use the word *cognition* to describe mental skills. Cognition includes understanding, reasoning, and gaining knowledge. Cognitive skills, like the motor and language skills discussed in Key 17, arise in a fairly typical pattern. For example, a child begins to imitate the actions of an adult before she learns object consistency or object permanence. Object permanence means a child understands that something still exists even if it is hidden. Before gaining this skill, a child will not look under a blanket for a hidden toy. After developing object permanence, a child learns causality or cause and effect. This means the child understands that when she does something, her action will make another thing happen. She knows that when she turns the crank, the jack-in-the-box will pop up. She begins to learn that if she touches something hot, it will hurt. Next, a child learns spatial relationships. She avoids obstacles when walking, places a toy on or under a chair on request, and learns the concepts of distance and size.

As with all developmental skills, age ranges act as guidelines of what to expect at certain stages. Milestones for cognitive development are listed in Table 2. These milestone ages are not the most important factor in mental development. Seeing your child progress from one stage to the next is important.

A child with cerebral palsy may not be able to meet many of these milestones on time because of poor movement or language skills. This does not necessarily mean that she has poor thinking skills as well. If your child is not excessively drowsy, pays attention to things going on around her, and makes facial expressions, you have some good clues about her intelligence.

In a child with cerebral palsy, intelligence may need to be tested in unique and unconventional ways that take into consideration the child's physical abilities and limitations. For example, a common test of object permanence is to see if a child picks up a toy she has dropped. This indicates she knows the toy still exists. If your child is unable to pick up an object, you would look to see if she indicated a desire for the object in another way such as making sounds when the object falls, looking for the object, and so on. Someone who knows your child well should help professionals when they test intelligence.

## YOUR CHILD'S MENTAL DEVELOPMENT

**Table 2**
**COGNITIVE MILESTONES**

| Age in Months | Skills |
|---|---|
| 0–2 | watches parent, quiets when held, responds to sounds, smiles, vocalizes, shows pleasure, shows interest in surroundings |
| 2–4 | inspects own hands, begins to play with rattles, imitates mouth movements |
| 4–6 | opens mouth when bottle or breast approaches, looks for dropped toy |
| 6–8 | imitates familiar gestures, finds hidden object, plays peekaboo, looks for family members when named |
| 8–10 | responds to *No*, moves to regain object and continues to play |
| 10–12 | imitates pat-a-cake, lifts arm or foot for dressing |
| 12–18 | laughs at funny actions, shows understanding of color, shows interest in books, identifies 1 body part |
| 18–24 | points to distant objects, matches sounds to animals, identifies 3 to 6 body parts |
| 24–30 | understands what some objects are used for, sorts by shapes, obeys two-part commands, plays simple make-believe activities |
| 30–36 | points to larger or smaller objects, plays house, sorts by color, completes simple jigsaw puzzles |

Sources: Ronald Illingworth, *The Development of the Infant and Young Child: Normal and Abnormal* (Edinburgh, Scotland: Churchill Livingston, 1987).

Setsu Furuno, *HELP Charts* (Palo Alto, CA: VORT Corp., 1994).

Some children with cerebral palsy who are very limited in movement skills may actually enjoy and be better at thinking skills. For example, a child with very stiff or spastic movements may have a long attention span and increased attention to details because mental activities are easier than physical activities.

Reading and listening to music may be more enjoyable and less frustrating than playing with toys. Finding an outlet for your child's thoughts and creativity is very important. For some children, using a computer with adaptive equipment allows their full intellectual potential to emerge. For others, learning sign language or using a communication board may work wonders. For many children whose language skills are impaired, frustration is a big issue. They have a lot to say but are unable to speak in conventional ways. If given an alternative way to communicate, many children can pleasantly surprise their parents by how much they actually know.

Whether or not your child has learning problems, you must teach her daily living skills such as dressing, bathing, using money, preparing meals, and following directions. These skills will allow her to be as independent as possible. They will help her become a contributing member of society by decreasing her reliance on others and increasing her ability to perform tasks that may lead to a job or other rewarding activities. Many times parents and teachers place so much emphasis on reading, writing, and arithmetic that they forget to teach skills to help children with cerebral palsy get through their everyday lives. Your child needs to receive teaching that is appropriate and most helpful to her instead of what is conventional or expected for her age or disability.

Unfortunately, in today's society, many people judge intelligence based on physical abilities. It is not uncommon to hear comments such as, "She is walking at nine months? She must be very smart." Therefore, when a child does not do what is physically expected at certain ages, people tend to assume she is not as smart as other children. This, of course, is completely untrue. Your child will progress at her own pace in mental development just as she does in all other areas of development. Always encourage your child and provide new learning opportunities to help her reach higher skills. You cannot completely predict how much your child will learn. However, she should always be given the opportunity to continue learning.

# 20

# YOUR CHILD'S SOCIAL DEVELOPMENT

Social development may begin before an infant is born. When tested, newborns consistently turn their faces toward their mother's voice at the time of birth. Perhaps the infant is listening to his mother's voice even before he is born. Social development typically follows a relatively predictable course.

In the first three months of life, children need a great deal of cuddling and contact. Socially, they begin to look at faces. They cry to signal their needs. Their cries become more specialized over time. Mothers can recognize one cry for hunger, another for pain, and another for boredom.

In the child with a damaged and immature brain, these steps may or may not proceed normally. The child may not look at his parents' faces. Instead of cuddling, the child may feel floppy or stiff. Instead of being awake, alert, and watchful for periods during the day, the child may sleep for very long periods of time. On the other hand, he may be very, very irritable and difficult to quiet. Bouts of crying can be long, loud, unpredictable, unusually high pitched, and very distressing for parents. Jerking, twitching, and trembling are often observed during crying. These babies are often described as *colicky*. The crying may be connected to how easily the child's immature nervous system is overloaded by lights, noises, sounds, movement, and daily activities.

In normal development at three to six months of age, the baby begins to have fewer bouts of unexplained crying. He recognizes his parents by sight, voice, smell, and touch. He begins to capture their attention by smiling and making cooing baby noises. The noises are mostly long chains of vowel sounds. He also begins to laugh. By the fifth month, the baby lifts up his arms to be held. The baby fusses when something happens that he does not like and makes happy noises when he likes something or someone. The baby frequently fusses in a strange situation or with a strange person.

For the three- to six-month-old child with cerebral palsy, social development may continue normally. On the other hand, the baby may have difficulty making eye contact and may stiffen his body when held. He may fail to make baby noises in response to his parents' coaxing and may not participate in pulling the corner of a blanket off his face to play peekaboo. Parents may wonder if the child is watching and recognizing them. Very irritable crying may be his only way to communicate.

For the infant with normal development, the six- to nine-month period is when he enjoys frolicking with parents and being thrown in the air or tickled. The baby shows increased anxiety when left with a stranger. He begins to smile and interact with his face in the mirror and to distinguish himself as separate from his mother.

The child with cerebral palsy may follow the same course, or he may continue to have great difficulty with social skills. His nervous system may continue to be very irritable and crying may still be his major method of communicating. He may still become easily upset and overloaded by ordinary daily events or changes in routine.

Typically, a nine to twelve month old imitates adults. He begins to put objects in and out of containers, learns new ways to play with toys, and begins to assert his opinion. He has definite likes and dislikes. He crawls, pulls up to stand, and walks while holding the furniture. He explores everything he can find and begins to have definite opinions about eating and bedtime.

Many children with cerebral palsy have difficulty moving into the normal developmental stage of exploring their environment. They may lack the movement skills to explore their surroundings or grasp things that they find. As a result, children with cerebral

## YOUR CHILD'S SOCIAL DEVELOPMENT

palsy, particularly those with lower intelligence, are more at risk for self-stimulating behaviors. Self-stimulation can include hand flapping, rocking, head banging, staring at lights, and hand biting. Children with cerebral palsy sometimes use these activities to calm themselves when stressed or overstimulated, or to entertain themselves when bored. These habits can interfere with their learning other, more appropriate skills.

Encourage your child to interact with people and explore his world. Interaction with caregivers and other children is crucial to social and mental development. Your child's ability to learn and socialize is related to his ability first to imitate and then to interact with the parent or caregiver. Encourage imitation, make sounds to your baby, encourage eye contact, listen quietly to your child, and respond to his sounds.

As your child grows older, the key to social development is interaction with other people, exploration of the environment, and playing. Parents need to understand that playing with other children is an opportunity to master important social skills. These include sharing, taking turns, using imagination, and gaining self-esteem. Your child's social development also largely depends on having frequent contact with friends, attending school regularly, and developing interests.

As your child enters the teenage years, he will face the same growing up issues all adolescents do. Trying to fit in with his peer group, self-image, independence from parents, self-consciousness, and developing attractions to the opposite sex are often very important issues for the adolescent. Your child may need extra support at this time because of the challenges his disability brings.

With sensitivity, you can help your child with cerebral palsy grow and develop socially. He deserves a life full of love, friends, and fun. He needs the opportunity to participate fully in family and community life.

# 21

# COMMON HEALTH PROBLEMS

Many children with cerebral palsy are perfectly healthy. They have only the usual illnesses of childhood. Cerebral palsy itself is not a progressive condition, and it does not cause a child to die. If other medical problems are well managed, your child will likely live a normal life span. However, certain predictable health problems are much more common in children with cerebral palsy.

Neurological problems or problems in brain function may be one of the earliest clues that a child has cerebral palsy. Seizures or convulsions occur in approximately 60 percent of children with cerebral palsy. Seizures are abnormal discharges of electrical activity in the brain. They cause a child to be unaware of what is going on around her. Some children have unusual jerks or twitches of body parts, unusual eye movements, or staring spells. Some seizures last only a few seconds, others last minutes or hours. Some children have difficulty breathing when they are having a seizure. You should call 911 immediately if your child has trouble breathing or looks blue during a seizure. Seizures are usually treated by a neurologist with medications. Seizure medications must be taken exactly as directed by your physician. Some seizure medications can cause side effects. Blood testing is required to make sure the medication is safe and effective. Some children outgrow their seizures as they become older. Other children have seizures throughout their lives. The goal is to control the seizures by making them less frequent and less intense so that a child's learning is not disrupted by them. Children with cerebral palsy can also have *hydrocephalus*, which occurs when fluid circulation inside the brain is partially or totally blocked. Hydrocephalus can result in an enlarged skull and brain damage. A shunt may be required to drain the fluid and protect the brain from additional damage.

Orthopedic problems with bones, muscles, and joints are very common. People with cerebral palsy are at risk of developing scoliosis, contractures, dislocated joints, and other deformities. These complications are discussed in more detail in Key 18.

Many children with cerebral palsy have difficulty eating and getting enough nutrition. Pediasure or other high-calorie supplements may be beneficial. Sometimes, feeding by mouth cannot be done safely or it takes too long to offer a child enough calories for growth. Refer to Key 23 for more information on feeding your child.

Other children with cerebral palsy are at risk of becoming dangerously overweight because they do not move around well. They just do not burn the number of calories that more active children do. Food intake should be carefully monitored. If a child becomes too heavy, her ability to move, transfer, or walk will suffer because of the increased demands on her body. An overweight child also places her parents at risk for back injuries.

Children with cerebral palsy are somewhat more prone to develop problems in the stomach and intestines as well. The digestive system is one continuous tube that runs from the child's mouth to the anus. Circular rings of muscles called sphincters close off sections of the digestive tract during various phases of digestion and keep the food moving in only one direction. Children with cerebral palsy are more likely to have poor coordination or sluggishness moving food through the digestive system. The smooth muscles of the digestive tract normally contract in waves called *peristalsis*. If peristalsis waves are too slow, gas, bloating, and constipation may result. Stomach acid may flow back into the food pipe called the esophagus if sphincters fail to close properly. This problem is called *gastroesophageal reflux*.

In addition to food moving slowly through the digestive tract, poor abdominal muscle tone and lack of upright positioning help cause constipation. Low fluid intake and a low-fiber diet are also often to blame. Children with cerebral palsy may have difficulty chewing the fruits, vegetables, and grains that would result in more regular, soft, comfortable stools. A physician can help develop a good bowel management program.

Breathing problems are also more common in children with cerebral palsy, especially infants who were born prematurely. A premature baby may require a machine called a ventilator to help her take breaths because her lungs can be very stiff, immature, and difficult to expand. When a mechanical ventilator helps with breathing for long periods of time, lung damage called *bronchopulmonary dysplasia* (BPD) may occur. When BPD happens, a child with cerebral palsy may continue to require oxygen or a mechanical ventilator only at night or up to twenty-four hours a day. As their lungs mature, many children no longer need oxygen or ventilation.

As a result of abnormal muscle tone and structure in the upper airway, some children have noisy, partially obstructed breathing called *stridor*. These children often sound like they are snoring or gasping even when their lungs are clear. Other children have difficulty remembering to breathe automatically. *Apnea* occurs when a child stops breathing for a few seconds. Usually, a child with apnea will begin to breathe again if gently jiggled or tapped. Some families use a monitor to sound an alarm if the child stops breathing. Some children with severe respiratory problems have a surgical opening in their windpipe called a *tracheostomy*, which allows them to breathe more safely. A ventilator may or may not be necessary in that case. The tracheostomy opening can be allowed to close and heal if the child can breathe safely without the opening.

Another common respiratory problem for children with cerebral palsy is *aspiration*—choking on saliva, food, or liquids and inhaling the material into the lungs. Inhaling anything into the lungs can cause pneumonia, a frequent reason children with cerebral palsy are admitted to the hospital. They may be more likely to contract pneumonia because of aspiration or perhaps because of more frequent colds and upper respiratory infections. Children with cerebral palsy often have a weak cough or pick up infections from other ill people, healthcare personnel, or medical equipment. A child who has a tracheostomy is much more likely to contract upper respiratory infections because germs have an easier route into the airway.

Some children with cerebral palsy are prone to skin problems. Wet diapers and frequent sitting can lead to rashes, infections, or pressure sores. Poor nutrition and being thin may lead to sores on bony parts like the tailbone, spine, hips, or heels. Unusual callouses may build up in odd places, like elbows, knees, feet, and ankles, where the child bears a great deal of weight. Wearing casts, braces, or splints can also lead to blisters or areas of open skin. If the child moves infrequently, she is at much higher risk for skin problems. Good positioning, keeping skin clean and dry, and frequent repositioning are keys to having healthy skin.

Urinary tract infections occur slightly more often in people with cerebral palsy. Not drinking enough fluids frequently causes the infection. Girls or women who have difficulty cleaning their skin well after a bowel movement may accidentally wipe bacteria from the rectum to the opening of the urinary tract, causing a urinary tract infection.

Another common problem is injury from falling. Children with cerebral palsy who are learning to sit or walk frequently fall down. Encourage your child's therapist to teach your child to fall safely. If your child has unpredictable falls and does not use her arms well enough to protect her head, a helmet may be necessary. Some of the most dangerous falls may occur if your child has a seizure while walking. During a seizure, she will be unable to protect her head because she is unconscious. A protective helmet may be recommended. If your child protects her head and face well when she falls and her injuries are limited to scratches and scrapes, a helmet may not be necessary. In that case, teach your child to stand up as independently as possible, reassure teachers and other caregivers, and keep both a supply of Band-Aids and a positive attitude. This will help increase your child's confidence. With the information from this key, you will be well informed about common health problems your child may face so you can better protect your child's health.

# 22
# VISION, HEARING, AND DENTAL CONCERNS

Vision problems are a concern for people with cerebral palsy. Muscle balance between the eyes may be poor; the eyes may appear to cross as they orient toward the bridge of the nose. *Strabismus* or crossing of the eyes can be treated by a combination of glasses, patches, eye exercises, and/or surgery. Another common and much more serious vision problem is *cortical visual impairment* or cortical blindness. With a cortical vision problem, the child's eye can take in light, but the electrical and chemical message that a visual image sends to the brain cannot be decoded. The child sees the equivalent of "snow" on a television screen.

Children with cerebral palsy, like other children, can have nearsightedness or farsightedness and may need corrective glasses. Children with brain damage may also have a visual field deficit in which they may not be able to see objects on one side, on the top, or on the bottom of the area being watched. To function better, the child may tilt her head sideways or turn her whole body slightly so that she can see a more complete spacial area. Prism glasses that capture the images in the problem visual field can help some people. A specialist in vision training at your child's school can teach your child to be more independent despite a visual impairment.

Some children with cerebral palsy have a hearing impairment. Some are completely deaf, while others may have some degree of hearing loss. Any child with a history of frequent ear infections may have some degree of hearing loss. A child who was exposed to a viral infection before birth may have a hearing impairment. A child

## VISION, HEARING, AND DENTAL CONCERNS

who developed an infection in the brain or coverings of the spinal cord after birth, like encephalitis or meningitis, may suffer a hearing loss or deafness. If wax, fluid, or other material blocks conduction of sound waves to the ear, a correctable hearing loss may result. Check with your child's doctor and audiologist if you suspect a hearing loss. Hearing aides may be prescribed. Some children with cerebral palsy have difficulty interpreting the meaning of sound in the brain, an auditory processing problem. When mild, the child has some difficulty differentiating between similarly sounding letters. When severe, it causes all sounds to seem mixed up and meaningless.

The teeth of some children with cerebral palsy may need special attention. Some antibiotics, such as tetracycline, can cause abnormalities in the hard white enamel covering of the teeth. Seizure medications can cause gums to grow more than their usual size and become thick, swollen, and prone to bleeding. Children with cerebral palsy may have irregularly spaced teeth or very small jaws that lead to tooth crowding and malalignment. Teeth may be cone shaped, of poor quality, or missing the protective enamel covering. Cavities are common because of difficulty brushing teeth well, poor enamel, and prolonged periods of time sucking from a bottle.

Armed with the information from this Key, you will be prepared to handle any special vision, hearing, or dental problems that your child with cerebral palsy might encounter. Your child's ability to see and hear are important for overall independence. Understanding visual, hearing, and dental problems can have an impact on your child's quality of life.

# 23

# HELPING YOUR CHILD TO EAT

One of the most common issues facing new parents is feeding. Parents of children both with and without cerebral palsy wonder: Is my child eating enough? Am I feeding him too often or not often enough? Does he eat too fast or too slow? Nothing can make a parent more worried than a child who will not or cannot eat. For many children with cerebral palsy, eating difficulties may be the first problem noticed. Difficulties include slow feeding, coughing, choking, or poor coordination. Some of these problems are easily corrected, while others require more intense interventions.

Quite often, children with cerebral palsy take a very long time to eat. This may mean an hour of breast-feeding or longer than thirty minutes to finish a bottle. Long feeding times have several possible causes. One is poor *oral motor* coordination. The child is unable to make the mouth, tongue, cheeks, and lips all work together to suck and swallow. Newborns usually have a pattern of suck-suck-swallow that gradually progresses to ten to fifteen sucks per swallow. If a child is unable to establish a rhythmical sucking and swallowing pattern he usually takes a long time to finish a small amount of liquid. A second reason for a prolonged feeding time may be a weak suck, where a child has difficulty forming a seal around the nipple. He only pulls a very small amount out with each suck.

One treatment for this problem is oral motor therapy. This teaches a child how to coordinate or strengthen the suck/swallow sequence. Oral motor therapy is usually performed by an occupational therapist or speech pathologist. If your child has been eating poorly for a while and his doctors are concerned with weight gain, tube feedings may be suggested to help meet nutritional needs while your child improves his eating skills. A tube feeding can consist of a nasogastic tube, which runs from the nose to the stomach, or an orogastric tube, which runs from the mouth to the stomach. These tubes are not permanent and can be removed after each feeding or when your child no longer needs them.

If your child coughs or chokes frequently when eating or drinking, he may have a common problem called *aspiration*. The swallowed food or liquid goes into the lungs instead of the stomach. Aspiration can be caused by poor coordination in the throat muscles used while swallowing. It can also result from food returning up from the stomach and then going into the windpipe and lungs. A possible solution is to thicken liquids. Thicker liquids travel through the mouth slower, allowing extra time to swallow safely. If this does not help, your child's therapist may experiment with different positions to use when feeding. Bringing the child's head forward and sitting him upright versus using a reclined position may reduce aspiration. If all attempts fail, your child is at risk for developing aspiration pneumonia. Tube feedings, oral motor therapy, and a swallow function study may be suggested. If aspiration occurs very frequently, a gastrostomy tube may be needed. This tube is surgically placed into the child's stomach to bypass the swallowing process. A gastrostomy tube is not necessarily permanent and may be removed if no longer needed.

Some newborns are unable to coordinate sucking, swallowing, and breathing. This usually results in longer feeding times with little food taken in and poor weight gain. Treatment may again include tube feedings to supplement nutrition as well as oral motor therapy to improve skills. *Nonnutritive sucking* uses a pacifier or a person's finger to help stimulate a coordinated pattern of sucking and breathing. No aspiration occurs because liquids and food are not swallowed. Often, a therapist can teach parents these techniques. Together, you can help your child gain the skills he lacks.

For older children who have difficulty chewing and swallowing, interventions are usually the same, including oral motor therapy and tube feedings, if necessary. Key 30 includes suggestions about dealing with gagging, tongue thrust or pushing food out with the tongue, and poor lip closure.

If your baby has a difficult time with eating, whether breastfeeding, bottle-feeding, or eating solids, talk with your child's doctor. The doctor can refer you to a therapist, dietician, or team of feeding specialists. They can develop a plan with you to best meet your child's physical, nutritional, and emotional needs.

One *very* important thing to know is that dealing with feeding issues can be a very slow, frustrating process. Feeding is much more complicated than most people realize and has a lot of emotional issues for both parents and children. Try your best not to become too overwhelmed. Expect to be frustrated at how long it takes to improve eating skills. Talk about your feelings with your child's team. Remember, they have been through this before and can help you get through it, too.

# 24

# WORKING WITH YOUR CHILD'S HEALTHCARE TEAM

When your child has cerebral palsy, you will suddenly find yourself meeting and working with a large group of medical professionals. As a parent, you will play perhaps the most important role on your child's healthcare team. You will choose most of the medical professionals who will work with your child. You will supply most of the information that the professionals need to provide their services. You will also share information about what other team members are working on with your child. Most parents find it very helpful to know who all these medical professionals are and what they do.

One of your first decisions will be to choose a primary care physician for your baby. A primary care physician will oversee your child's general healthcare and make referrals to other doctors. Ideally, your child's primary care physician will be a pediatrician. A pediatrician is a physician who specializes in providing medical care for children.

If your child was born prematurely or had medical complications at the time of birth that were serious enough for him to be cared for in a neonatal intensive care unit, then your child's primary care physician may be a neonatologist. A neonatologist is a pediatrician who specializes in the care of seriously ill or high-risk newborns. When your child moves past the newborn stage, a general pediatrician will usually take over, especially after a child is discharged from the hospital.

Other specializing physicians may be consulted to look at or assist in managing a particular type of health problem. A neurologist evaluates brain function and treats seizures. A neurosurgeon handles any necessary brain surgery and may also perform a surgery to reduce spasticity. An orthopedist deals with problems of bones, joints, or muscles and performs surgery on them, if necessary. Through yearly checkups, the orthopedic deformities related to cerebral palsy may be managed or avoided. A gastroenterologist may be consulted for any digestive problems your child has such as vomiting his feedings or gastroesophageal reflux, a common complication. A urologist may be needed to manage issues related to the kidneys, bladder, and urination. This doctor can prescribe medication to treat urinary tract infections and prevent bladder spasms. The urologist may design a bladder training program to help with incontinence, resulting in fewer accidents and staying drier.

A developmental pediatrician has additional expertise in children with developmental delays or disabilities. A physical medicine physician, sometimes called a physiatrist, specializes in working with children with disabilities like cerebral palsy. A physical medicine physician can fully evaluate your child and direct a comprehensive inpatient or outpatient rehabilitation program. This may include medication, therapy, bracing, splinting, casting, or special equipment. A physical medicine physician may also perform special diagnostic tests such as nerve conduction velocity testing or electromyography.

If your child needs help with behavioral issues, you may work with a psychiatrist, psychologist, or neuropsychologist. A neuropsychologist deals with behavioral issues in people who have some problem with brain function. A psychiatrist is a medical doctor who may prescribe medication or other treatments to address behavioral or emotional issues. A psychologist is a professional member of the mental healthcare team who may counsel a patient with cerebral palsy or his family. A psychologist may assist in designing and implementing a behavior management program.

## WORKING WITH YOUR CHILD'S HEALTHCARE TEAM

Your child may work with nurses, nurse's aides, or personal care attendants. Registered nurses and licensed practical nurses will take care of your child when hospitalized. They may provide nursing support in your home or child's school. They also supervise nurse's aides or personal care attendants who have received classroom instruction and on-the-job training to assist in your child's care in the home. Home care is discussed in Key 31.

Physical therapists and physical therapy assistants are primarily concerned with developing your child's independent movement skills and preventing orthopedic complications. Occupational therapists and occupational therapy assistants teach "occupations" of daily living. For a child, these include playing, eating, bathing, going to school, dressing, and more. An occupational therapist may concentrate on fine motor skills, academic skills, or preparation for job training. Speech language pathologists may play a role in your child's feeding program and will be primarily concerned with his ability to communicate. The speech pathologist may concentrate on improving verbal speech and teaching other forms of communication. Please refer to Key 25 for further information on therapy.

With so many people involved in your child's care, confusion and frustration are common for both parents and professionals. For that reason, it is important for parents to identify a case manager to organize and coordinate all of their child's services. Your child's case manager will usually be a social worker but can be a parent, rehabilitation counselor, medical professional, or nonlicensed person. A case manager is someone very familiar with your child's needs. This person has an excellent working knowledge of all the programs and services available to meet your child's needs. It is vitally important that a single person carefully follow your child's progress and participate in all program changes. This allows a single person to see the big picture of your child. Most social programs and some insurance companies provide case managers for their clients. Parents should make sure that whoever serves as case manager knows their child very well, is very knowledgeable about resources, is very diplomatic, and puts their child's needs first. The case manager should not be concerned only with saving money for an insurance company or program.

# 25

# WHAT IS THERAPY?

Most parents of a child with cerebral palsy will, at some time, come into contact with one type of therapist or another. Many times, these therapists become an important part of the child's life. The time line for when a child begins or ends therapy depends on each child's individual needs.

The most common types of therapy involve occupational therapists, physical therapists, or speech language pathologists. Each type of therapy has its areas of specialty, but much overlap occurs among the groups. In general, these professionals work together to address your child's overall physical, mental, social, and functional skill development.

Occupational therapists usually concentrate on the areas of fine motor skills or hand/finger coordination, feeding, arm functioning, cognitive development, and overall developmental skills. Activities of daily living such as dressing, cooking, and bathing are stressed. Visual/perceptual skills, which include identifying and recognizing letters and shapes, are also addressed by occupational therapists.

Physical therapists usually concentrate on gross motor skills such as sitting, crawling, walking, and running. They help a child learn how to move from one position to another. Physical therapists emphasize activities to improve strength, balance, flexibility, endurance, coordination, and overall developmental skills.

Speech language pathologists work on speech and language skills, swallowing difficulties, and, sometimes, feeding issues. They emphasize communication and oral motor skills. Often, they work with audiologists to test and treat a child's hearing problems.

## WHAT IS THERAPY?

Some physical, occupational, or speech therapists have additional training or special certification that may be very helpful for your child with cerebral palsy. A certified neurodevelopmental therapist has completed an extensive training program on treatment techniques specifically designed for children with cerebral palsy. Neurodevelopmental treatment (NDT) focuses on promoting normal or more functional movement patterns. A certified sensory integration therapist has received additional training in a therapeutic technique that stresses the importance of how the child's brain processes touch, balance, and other sensory information. Sensory integration (SI) may be very helpful in improving your child's coordination, writing skills, attention span, and many other areas.

Other types of therapy that your child may receive at some point include recreation therapy, music therapy, hippotherapy, and art therapy. Recreation therapists involve people with disabilities in recreational and leisure activities ranging from a game of solitaire to attending sporting events. Emphasis is placed on teaching people to make choices, develop interests, and make friends. A recreation therapist may also teach someone how to participate in recreation and leisure activities in the community. Examples include using public transportation to go to the mall, obeying traffic signs when riding a bike, and planning a trip. Your child's regular or adapted physical education teacher may also have suggestions for recreation activities you can do at home.

Music therapy, like recreation therapy, is often available at treatment centers or places where many people with disabilities live. Music therapists use all forms of music to address some of the same goals as recreation therapy. Music can also promote relaxation or improve motivation. Shaking a tambourine or playing a drum can be good exercise, too. Hippotherapy, or horseback riding therapy, is available in many communities and is very beneficial for children with cerebral palsy. The rhythmic movement of the horse, specific exercises, and the emotional bond between the child and the horse can be very therapeutic. Art therapy may be available in various forms. The performing arts and creative arts give a person a form of expression. They can enhance movement, socialization, and communication skills and can increase confidence.

The goals of therapy are to help your child become as functional, independent, and self-fulfilled as possible. Therapy may be provided in groups or on an individual basis. Usually, therapists will evaluate your child the first time they see her to determine what skills she is able to do and in what areas she needs some extra help. Once an evaluation has been completed, it is time to develop goals. Discuss your priorities for your child with the therapist so that you can develop realistic goals together. If you think eating and crawling are the most important issues, tell your child's therapists so they can work with you to achieve these goals as well as any goals the child wants to work on.

The number of weekly therapy sessions and the length of the sessions vary depending on the child's needs and the setting. Most therapists will use toys and games to engage your child in an activity. At times, the therapists may choose to work together with your child to achieve particular goals.

You will play a very important role in therapy. Learning how to handle or move your child in certain ways to help her learn to move better will be one way you can practice new skills at home. A home program can include many different activities and ideas. Try to be very involved in your child's therapy sessions. Get in there and do the activities with the therapists. Ask them what they are doing and why. This will help you to carry out the home program. Therapy can be both rewarding and helpful, but it is also time consuming. Always relate how you are feeling about what is going on with your child to the therapists so they can make things go more smoothly for you and attempt to achieve your child's goals.

# 26

# NEW TRENDS IN MEDICAL MANAGEMENT

Improvements are being made in medication, surgery, therapy, and equipment to treat cerebral palsy. Children with cerebral palsy can look forward to better control of seizures with fewer side effects than ever before. New seizure medications and new combinations of medications allow children to have fewer seizures with less disruption of their ability to concentrate and learn.

New medications are available that help reduce drooling. A dental device that improves swallowing through better lip closure and surgery on the salivary glands are other options to reduce drooling. Medication may also help children who have short attention spans concentrate on what they are doing. Medications such as Valium or Bacloflen are being used by children with cerebral palsy to help relax very stiff and tight muscles.

Some children use a *Baclofen pump* to treat their spasticity. The Bacloflen pump is surgically placed under the skin of the back very near the spinal cord. It releases tiny amounts of Bacloflen to help relax tightness or spasticity at the spinal cord level. Once the spasticity decreases, the child should be more comfortable and have improved abilities. The child must be thoroughly evaluated to determine if the benefits of a Bacloflen pump are worth the risks of surgery.

A medication called Botulinum toxin can be injected directly into a tight muscle to help reduce its abnormal muscle tone. While the muscle is temporarily relaxed, the body part can be casted to improve its alignment. The cast takes advantage of this relaxation and stretches tight muscles. Botulinum toxin can also help a child benefit more from a therapy program. Botulinum toxin only relaxes a muscle temporarily. A great deal of effort and therapy must be given to strengthen surrounding muscles to achieve better function. Your child's body weight affects how many muscles can be treated with Botulinum toxin and how much can be used. Botulinum toxin is relatively expensive and its effects are temporary, usually lasting about three months. Therefore, its use should be targeted for a particular problem, well planned, and timed to address growth spurts.

A select number of children with cerebral palsy may benefit from a neurological operation for managing spasticity. *Selective dorsal rhizotomy* is a major surgical procedure where the backbone is surgically opened with an operation called a laminectomy. Next, the spinal cord and its nerve roots are exposed. The sensory roots of the spinal cord are then gently stimulated electrically one at a time. If a movement is more abnormal and spastic with stimulation, the surgeon may cut that particular tiny root, thus reducing the amount of spasticity. This is a major, permanent surgical procedure. Once sensory nerve roots to the spinal cord are cut, they will never work again. Recovery from this surgery requires months of very intensive physical and occupational therapy. The ultimate results of the surgery cannot be exactly predicted beforehand. The skill and prior experience of the surgeon is of the utmost importance. The child is evaluated by a team of specialists to determine if the child is a good candidate for the procedure.

Advances in casting and splinting are also helping to prevent contracture, improve posture and tone, and improve use of body parts. Physicians, physical therapists, and occupational therapists frequently make casts or splints. A cast or splint can be *serial*, which means it is adjusted or replaced several times in order to lengthen shortened tissue gradually. A cast or splint can be *inhibitive*, which means it supports or creates a body posture that reduces abnormal muscle tone or spasticity. Some casts and splints do both.

## NEW TRENDS IN MEDICAL MANAGEMENT

Braces called *orthotics* are better designed to help children with cerebral palsy than ever before. Orthotics are made of stronger, more durable, and lighter weight material. They are custom designed, molded, and fitted by medical professionals called orthotists. Orthotists work closely with your child's physician and therapist to design a brace that improves the posture and use of a body part. Orthotists can design braces to support any body part including the trunk, wrist, or ankle.

Surgeries are safer and offer greater improvement in positioning and function to children with cerebral palsy than ever before. Orthopedic surgery can improve curvature of the spine, hip dislocation, abnormal position of a limb, or shortened muscles. Parents should look for orthopedic surgeons who are experienced in operating on children with cerebral palsy.

Electrical stimulation is a treatment method that uses an electrical stimulator powered by a nine-volt battery. Electrodes are placed on the child's skin over specific muscles. A tiny amount of electrical current that causes a tickling, tapping, or twitch sensation is applied through the surface of the skin to stimulate muscles. In some children, the current may help relax tight muscles. The tickling or tapping sensation sometimes helps children to contract and control their muscles better. When the current causes the muscles to twitch or contract, strengthening occurs. Electrical stimulation should always be comfortable for the child and can be performed daily at home by the parents. The electrodes and stimulator are the size of a transistor radio and can be worn while the child walks, plays, or watches television. Some electrical stimulation programs use levels of current so low that the child cannot feel it.

*Biofeedback* is another treatment being explored to improve the movement control of children with cerebral palsy. A sensor is placed on the child's body. When the child performs a desired movement, such as tightening or relaxing a specific muscle, a signal is given. The signal can be a light, a sound, or even a picture or graph on a computer screen. Each time the child performs correctly, he hears a sound or sees a light or picture. Eventually, the child learns how to control the muscle or body function without the signal.

Many advances have been made in the management of other common health problems mentioned in Key 21. Due to these improvements, most children with cerebral palsy are able to live at home successfully, leading healthier and more productive lives.

# PART FIVE

# RAISING A CHILD WITH CEREBRAL PALSY

This part contains many useful suggestions for raising your child. Key 28 offers practical ideas for organizing for success. This includes using a care notebook, which gives other people tips about caring for your child. Part Five shares strategies for teaching your child to play. It also shows ways that children with cerebral palsy can help care for themselves to the best of their abilities. You will learn about programs to increase training opportunities. Part Five also assists you in dealing with your child's behavior.

# 27

# WHAT CAN WE EXPECT?

Two burning questions are on the minds of parents of a child with cerebral palsy: How will our child progress? and What can we expect? As with other children, you can expect your child to progress at her own individual rate. Children with cerebral palsy may have normal development in some areas and severe delays in other areas. For example, one child may be unable to roll over or sit up and yet can think and talk normally. Another child may walk without help but does not speak or seem to be aware of her surroundings.

The location, type, and extent of the brain damage can be a partial predictor of what to expect. However, some children with very severe disabilities have CT scans and MRIs that appear completely normal. Other children who are missing parts of the brain or have areas of severe damage function very well. Remember that CT scans and MRIs only look at the structure of the brain. They cannot measure how well an area of the brain works. Professionals who work with large numbers of children with cerebral palsy find that they can expect some common patterns of progression based mostly on the child's type of cerebral palsy.

Most children with cerebral palsy will have some abnormal patterns of movement that last throughout their lifetimes. As discussed in the Keys about development in Part Four, most children with cerebral palsy will be slower than other children to achieve their motor milestones. Depending on the extent of the brain damage, abnormal muscle tone, and abnormal reflexes, many children with cerebral palsy will "get stuck" at a particular point in the developmental progression and may fail to move beyond it. Sadly, some children get stuck in the very beginning stages of learning to move and have tremendous difficulty with simple skills like holding up their heads and holding onto toys. A child with cerebral palsy who struggles to move may use an abnormal reflex pattern on purpose just to create the power to complete the job. Predictably, this child will have difficulty learning a more normal movement pattern because the reflex pattern seems easier.

In some cases, premature babies who experience normal brain development before an early birth progress better than children with cerebral palsy who are born on time or late. Children who are born at term or later may have had abnormal brain development early in the pregnancy or throughout the pregnancy. They may never have experienced normal movement even in the womb.

The type of muscle tone your child has can help shape what to expect as your child develops. Children with hypotonia, without spasticity or seizures, often very slowly gain relatively normal movement skills. With therapy and practice, they learn to overcome their low tone, though they may tend to be uncoordinated. Children with hemiplegia will eventually walk, usually with a limp. They will have the greatest problems using the involved hand. The hand impairment can be mild or severe. Children with very mild diplegia typically walk with an unusual movement pattern. Children with moderate diplegia may walk short distances with braces, crutches, or walkers. They can usually use their hands pretty well. Children with spastic quadriplegia tend to have the most difficulty with movement. They get stuck more easily and have the greatest degree of developmental delay.

Predictably, as children with cerebral palsy become older and heavier, they are more likely to develop orthopedic problems. Scoliosis, dislocations, and contractures often develop as children grow older. Most of these problems can be well managed if followed closely and treated aggressively.

Other important factors can help predict how your child will progress. Hand and arm strength and function are critical for a child learning to walk with a walker or crutches and learning to dress or bathe herself. A child's opportunity to practice movement can strongly influence progress. Your child's thinking skills, vision, hearing, and seizure control can greatly influence how well and how quickly she develops. Children who can see and process visual information well are often highly motivated to get up and move toward toys or people they enjoy. Children who are ill, who have more severe intellectual problems, or whose learning is constantly interrupted by seizures have greater difficulties moving and learning. Intelligence, motivation, determination, and practice allow many children with cerebral palsy to do amazing things.

Many children with cerebral palsy have hidden talents that are unrecognized because most tests of intelligence depend on movement skills and speech. Perhaps an often overlooked barometer of true intelligence is a child's desire to explore her environment. Faster overall progress is usually made in children who try to explore their environment by looking at objects, making sounds to attract attention, and batting at or scooting toward a desired toy. Children who are caught in their own world of rocking, head banging, and flapping their hands typically progress much more slowly. These children need extensive therapy and home training to help develop exploration of the world outside themselves. Adapted switches and computers help improve a child's participation in the world. Remember that many children with severe physical disabilities are intelligent, and many children with self-stimulating behaviors just need a way to communicate. The challenge to parents is to unlock that potential.

If your child with cerebral palsy is not given opportunities to learn or try, you cannot expect her to improve. It is important to understand that learning any method for communication, such as pointing at pictures or using switches, may help to develop speaking skills. Simple movement, such as bouncing, swinging, and physical play, may stimulate the production of sound or speech. Learning any method of getting around, such as rolling, crawling, using a scooter board, or using a wheelchair, may encourage more independent walking in some children. Allow a child who uses a wheelchair lots of practice at walking or standing. Typical walking and talking may not be possible, but you never know what your child will learn if given a chance.

WHAT CAN WE EXPECT?

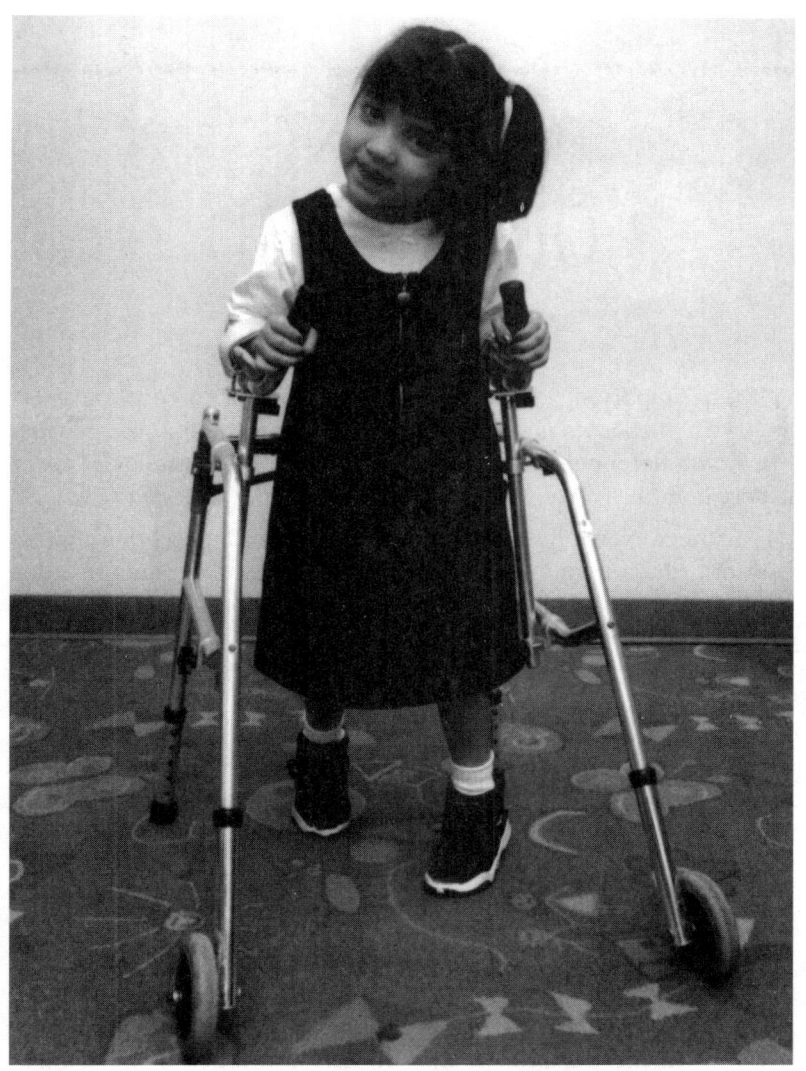

**Walking with my rolling walker**

# 28

# GETTING ORGANIZED

One important key to helping your child with cerebral palsy do his best is *getting organized*. Constructing a large loose-leaf notebook with several sections and a clear plastic cover is very helpful. The notebook becomes your child's *care notebook*.

You can have many sections in your child's notebook. In one section, place a calendar to keep track of appointments. Keep another section for all the special therapies or programs your child attends.

Keep a section for your child's complete medical records, including birth history, immunization records, reports from all the specialists your child has seen, and copies of all prescriptions for medications, therapy, or special equipment. Keep a section to list the names, specialties, addresses, and phone and fax numbers of all the providers who work with your child. You can add their business cards to this section. Keep your listings current. Save old listings because you may want to recontact that provider in the future for records or information.

In another section, keep a list of the dates, lengths of time, and names of the providers for all of your child's services. This is useful information in case any billing errors occur. Insurance, Medicare, or Medicaid information should have a section as well. Insurance cards, letters of authorization, and other payment information can be kept in this section.

An additional section can be added for each of your child's developmental tasks. One section should be titled "The Way I Like to Eat." It can contain any special diet, nutrition, or feeding instructions, and the preferred texture of your child's food. It can also list any food allergies, food likes, and food dislikes. It can describe the times, methods, and amounts for tube feeding.

Another notebook section can be titled "The Way I Like to Exercise." Your child's home exercise program, possibly including drawings or Polaroid pictures of any special equipment your child uses to exercise, should be included here. Additional sections in the care notebook might be, "How I Like to Get Dressed," "Where I Go to School," "How I Like to Be Positioned," "How I Communicate," and "Toys I Like to Play With."

Another section should be included called "My Friends and Family." Include names, addresses, and phone numbers of all parents and guardians. Pictures of family, friends, and pets that are special to your child with a description of each should be included. This lets professionals who work with your child know who is important to your little one.

You can add as many sections to this care notebook as you like. Insert your child's picture or artwork inside the front plastic cover. Make sure the notebook always accompanies your child. You can photocopy documents out of the notebook for professionals that need copies. You should keep original documents in a safe place in case the notebook is lost. The care notebook will be a big help in getting you organized to care for your child with cerebral palsy, but there are several other helpful tips as well.

If you are meeting with a service provider, write down all your questions ahead of time. This will help keep you on track and prevent forgetting an important question. Call the provider's office ahead of time to let the provider know what topic you want to discuss. A longer appointment time may be allowed for more discussion. The provider will also appreciate the chance to gather information and be better prepared for your questions.

Never be afraid to gather resources about your child's cerebral palsy or possible treatments yourself. If you find an article or program you are interested in, give a copy of the literature to your child's providers. They will probably be very eager to receive the latest information and help you evaluate it.

In organizing to best care for your child with cerebral palsy, know your child and family's rights and responsibilities. Your child has certain rights and responsibilities as a special education student, as a medical patient, and as a client of any special program in which he participates. Parents who understand their rights and responsibilities can receive the best treatment available from any program in which their child participates.

Conferences and meetings with healthcare professionals or school personnel will occur frequently. The information exchanged will be important to your child's progress. Never hesitate to bring a support person to a meeting or conference to help you feel more comfortable when you meet with these busy professionals. A support person can remind you of any questions you have forgotten to ask, provide emotional support, and help you listen, understand, and remember what the professionals said during the conference. The support person should take notes during the conference that you can read later.

A parent who has difficulty understanding, speaking, reading, or writing English should always try to bring a support person who can translate and perhaps assist in reading and filling out forms. You can call ahead and ask if a translator can be provided, but sometimes translators are not available. Many parents are more comfortable with a translator who is a friend or relative.

Always arrange to have a baby-sitter for all your children, including your child with cerebral palsy, when you need to meet for a formal conference with your child's service provider. It is impossible for parents to focus on the conversation if they have to handle fussy or noisy children. When possible, have a baby-sitter care for brothers and sisters at home. If the service provider needs to examine your child with cerebral palsy and then meet with you for discussion afterward, bring a responsible teenager or another adult with you who can supervise your child while you meet with the professionals. Arranging for day care ahead of time helps keep

## GETTING ORGANIZED

you from feeling frustrated when you need to focus on and fully participate in the important planning occurring for your child. Personal attendants or home health nurses can often help. On the other hand, remember that your child needs to be involved in planning his future. The attendant could assist your child in the meeting so that you can concentrate.

An important way to become organized is to register your child well in advance for programs you want to participate in now and in the future. Many programs are expensive. Funding assistance is available, but waiting lists are often very long. Processing new applications is often a lengthy process. Ask other parents, case managers, and your child's providers for guidance in this area.

An important program to help you become organized for the unpredictable emergencies in life is a good respite program. Find and enroll your child in a quality respite program as near to your home as possible. Keep your child's application, immunization records, and medical records current at the respite program in case of emergency.

When you are organizing to care for your child with cerebral palsy successfully, remember to plan ahead, but do not waste energy with fruitless worrying. If you have a concern or a worry, turn it into an *action plan*. Investigate resources and make phone calls. If you need help, *ask for it*. If a person will not help, ask someone else. With a little organization and planning, caring for the needs of your child with cerebral palsy can be a smoother, more rewarding experience. Through organization, parents often experience personal growth and achievement as they master the challenge of raising a child with cerebral palsy.

# 29

# TEACHING YOUR CHILD TO PLAY

Although play is a difficult word to define, most people know what it means. Play is the way children learn about the world around them. Play is important. It helps improve physical skills as well as develop thinking and social skills. It teaches about rules and working together, and it encourages imagination.

Often, a child with cerebral palsy does not play as much as other children, for many reasons. First, a lot of time is spent teaching the child to move, talk, and eat. Playing just to have fun is often overlooked. Another reason is that the child may find it difficult to hold and use toys in the usual way. The child who has trouble holding or picking up objects may have difficulty playing with many toys sold in stores. Finally, there may be a lack of time available to allow a child to play when medical needs seem to take up every minute of the day.

One way to help make play easier for your child is by adapting toys. Using Velcro or a sticky substance called Dycem can help a child pick up and hold onto toys. Making pieces of toys bigger and easier to hold can also be fairly simple and helpful. Adding switches to battery-powered toys is a very common way to help children with cerebral palsy control and operate toys and household objects. Ask your child's therapist for suggestions. Some of the assistive technology resources at the end of this book may also be helpful.

# TEACHING YOUR CHILD TO PLAY

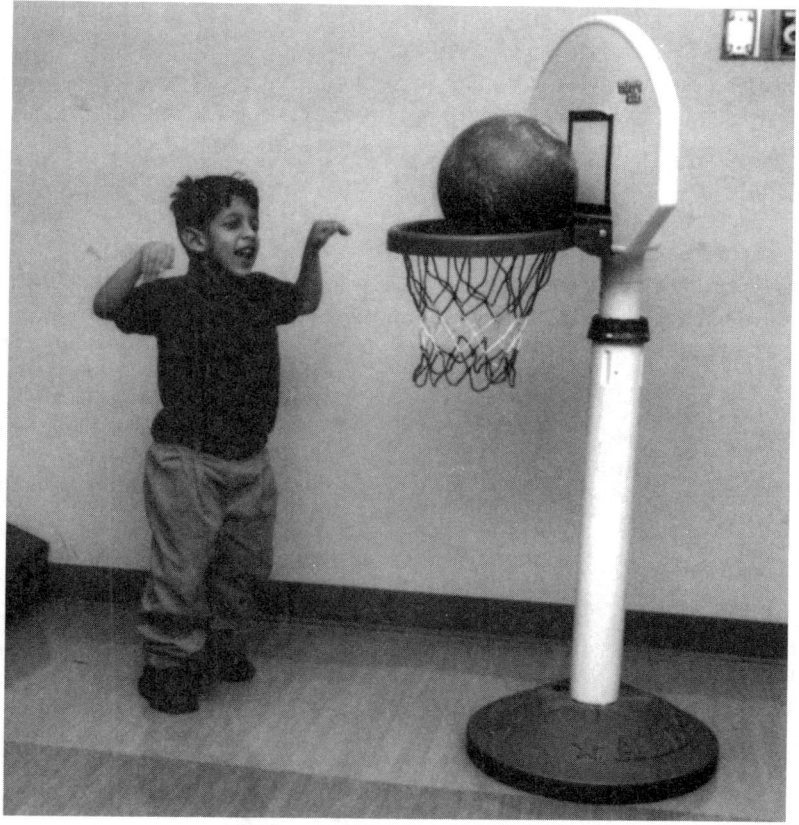

**I love to play basketball.**

Allowing children to play on their own is very important. Learning about the child's surroundings needs to be spontaneous and self-directed to help increase thinking skills and independence. By placing your child in a position that allows free use of her hands without having to work on sitting balance or head control, you can encourage and enable more independent play. Another important part of play is variety. Children lose interest quickly and require many different toys and activities to stay interested and excited. To keep your child interested, try to use several different play activities to practice one skill. For example, to teach shapes, use shape boxes, drawing shapes, finger painting, puzzles, and matching games. If your child has a problem with one of her senses, such as hearing or sight, you will need to help her learn and play with a different sense. For example, in a child who cannot see, using sound and touch will help teach her about the world. Toys that have sound and many different textures are best. If both sight and hearing are affected, using touch and movement can be added to teach a child about objects and having fun. Some toys that involve touch are pom-poms, play dough, sand, and a touch-and-feel book. Cloth scraps, carpet scraps, yarn, foil, and wrapping paper are also interesting to play with and touch.

The most important thing to remember when playing with your child is no matter what, play should be fun and safe. Play for children with special needs includes many activities and is restricted only by the limits of creativity.

# 30

# HELPING YOUR CHILD BECOME INDEPENDENT

It is very natural to want to help a child to dress, eat, and take a bath. Unfortunately, many times people assume that children with disabilities need help without checking to see if this is true. The best way to help your child develop self-care skills and become independent is to let him do as much for himself as possible.

For example, when taking off your child's shirt, leave it halfway on his head and let him pull it off. This not only increases independence and self-esteem but is also a good exercise for the arms. Children with cerebral palsy will be able to participate at different levels. Some children will become completely independent, and others may always need assistance. What is important is to let your child do as much as possible for himself, even if it is as simple as pushing his arm through a sleeve or pulling down his pants to use the bathroom.

One of the most common problems for children with cerebral palsy is eating. Your child may have trouble chewing, have trouble keeping his lips closed, gag on foods, or push food out of his mouth with his tongue. By changing the texture of food, many of these problems can be reduced. Food textures include runny, smooth, lumpy, chunky, chewy, and others. Methods to change food texture include mashing it with a fork, putting it into a blender, or making food or liquids thicker.

Cleanliness is another area of self-care that may require some creative adaptations to make your child feel independent. Using bath chairs or even an inner tube in the tub can help with sitting balance. Independence in bathing and hygiene can really improve a child's self-esteem.

Supportive positioning is extremely important in all areas of self-care for a person with cerebral palsy. Sitting on a firm seat with his feet on the floor can make a tremendous difference in how well a child eats, brushes his teeth, or folds his clothes. Without proper support, your child may not be able to do anything by himself.

Below are some basic hints for dressing, eating, and simple hygiene. Ask your child's therapists for specific ideas to increase your child's independence in these and other areas of self-care. Some of the assistive technology resources in the appendix have catalogs of equipment for self-care and positioning. Some of the listed suggested readings and a resource called Physiological Corporation provide valuable information on teaching independence.

**Dressing**
1. If your child can only use one arm and/or leg, have him dress the affected arm or leg first and undress it last.
2. You can make buttoning easier by using Velcro. Place the hook portion behind the buttons and the latch portion over the holes. This gives the appearance of a shirt with regular buttons, but increases the ease of dressing and undressing. Velcro can also take the place of zippers or shoelaces.
3. Use the technique of backward chaining to teach dressing. Teach the last step first. Once it is mastered, move to the next step. Steps to learn how to take off a shirt would be
   Step 1 Parent raises shirt to child's forehead and then the child pulls shirt off head by himself.
   Step 2 Child pulls arms out of shirt and then pulls shirt over head.
   Step 3 Child pulls bottom of shirt up, takes arms out, and pulls it off his head.
4. Use dress up games for practice.

## Eating

1. If your child has a hard time making the transition from baby foods or pureed foods to foods with texture or lumps, add a graham cracker to smooth, pureed food. At first, add mashed graham cracker. Slowly increase the size of the cracker pieces in the pureed food as tolerated, over time.
2. If your child tends to bite down on the spoon and is unable to release it, try to feed him by placing food in the sides of his mouth rather than the front. This problem can be caused by the tonic bite reflex, which is set off by touching the front teeth and causes an involuntary closing of the jaw or bite.
3. If your child is just learning to drink from a cup and liquids come out too fast, you can add baby cereal or Thick and Easy to thicken the liquid.
4. If your child pushes food out of his mouth with his tongue, press downward on his tongue with the spoon each time you offer a bite of food. You can also place your thumb under his chin for support to help keep his mouth closed and the tongue from coming forward. This problem is called tongue thrust.
5. Special equipment can be used to help your child feed himself. Utensils, plates, cups, and cookware can be purchased or adapted to allow more independence in eating and cooking.
6. Use pretend play such as tea parties to practice skills.

## Cleanliness

1. If your child has a hard time holding onto a washcloth, he can use a wash mitt. This is a glove that fits over the hand and can be used like a washcloth.
2. If your child is able to grasp only large or wide objects, build up the handles of toothbrushes or hairbrushes with rubber or foam tubing.
3. For children who are unable to sit independently or require a lot of assistance, various bath chairs are available to make this task easier.
4. Use dolls to practice appropriate hygiene skills. A fun play activity is giving a doll a bath.

# 31

# HOME CARE AND HABILITATION TRAINING

As a parent, you have many responsibilities. Having a child with cerebral palsy greatly increases the demands on your time. Not only are you responsible for your child's health, safety, and nurturing, you also have to find time to teach your child how to do things on her own. Home care and habilitation training are options that may be available to you. These services are provided to those who qualify. They reinforce or enhance the training your child receives from her family and therapists.

Although the name of the service varies from state to state, you can use the terms *home care* or *habilitation training* to receive more information from your child's case manager or your state's Departments of Health or Human Services. To habilitate means to give someone the ability to do something they could not do before. Through habilitation, a person with cerebral palsy learns how to perform a task on her own or to the best of her abilities. Home care and habilitation training provide this instruction to a child in her home.

*Rehabilitation,* which means relearning a lost skill, is a word you will encounter more often than habilitation. It describes therapy services and equipment used by people who have cerebral palsy. A person who has had a stroke may need rehabilitation in order to regain skills. Although habilitation is usually a more

## HOME CARE AND HABILITATION TRAINING

appropriate term for training someone who has cerebral palsy, you will probably find this term used only to describe services like the ones discussed in this Key.

Like respite care, as mentioned in Key 14, home care aides, habilitation training specialists, or personal care attendants are specially trained to work with people who have disabilities. They provide training in daily living skills like dressing, bathing, toileting, and so on. They can help with therapy after receiving instruction from your child's therapist. They can help your older child to prepare for and live independently by teaching skills like washing laundry and paying bills. The aide may also support your child and family by doing some housework, running errands, and providing stress relief. Sometimes, an additional person will perform these chores. Homemakers, as these aides are called, are usually available in group homes or shared living arrangements.

An aide, specialist, or attendant is supervised by the training agency, case manager, and family. Usually, an individualized habilitation plan (IHP) is written by your child's team. The IHP specifies the skills that need to be developed, and how and when the training will occur. Refer to Key 38 for details on IHPs. Besides contacting your state Department of Health or referring to this book's resource section, you may also find home care providers by talking with other parents of children with disabilities.

# 32

# MANAGING BEHAVIOR AND DISCIPLINE

A common misunderstanding is that children with disabilities *cannot* and *should not* be disciplined, that they should not be held accountable for their behavior. This could not be further from the truth. Most children with cerebral palsy who have a problem behavior are capable of having that problem behavior lovingly shaped into a more acceptable one.

Most children, even children who cannot speak, benefit from having a consistent, logical, calm, predictable consequence to their problem behavior. For example, a child with cerebral palsy who bites his hand might experience the consequence of being firmly told "no," having the bitten hand placed in a protective splint, and having his favorite music turned off for three minutes. Learning consequences of behavior and mastering behavioral control are chances for the child to improve his thinking skills and have greater opportunity to learn, work, and play with others.

Some of the special needs of a child with cerebral palsy may make problem behavior more likely and more frequent than with other children. Self-injurious behavior occurs when a child hits, bites, or scratches himself. Some children may hit their heads on the floor. Self-stimulating behavior may include shaking his head or hands, pressing on eye sockets, making noises, and rocking. Self-injurious or self-stimulating behaviors are seen more frequently in children with severe mental retardation or sensory impairments. It is important for a parent to look for what *triggers* whining, aggression, hurting himself, or a tantrum in a child. Problem behaviors have many common triggers.

## MANAGING BEHAVIOR AND DISCIPLINE

A child with cerebral palsy may physically or mentally tire more quickly. If pushed to the point of fatigue, problem behaviors may result. The solution is often as simple as some quiet time or a nap.

Children with cerebral palsy sometimes have difficulty processing sensory information. Loud noise, crowds, crying babies, bright colors, flickering lights, scratchy clothing, or unusual food textures may trigger crying or tantrums. Removing the trigger or the child from the overstimulating environment may stop the behavior. It is not unusual for these children to have tantrums during holiday gatherings, birthday parties, or while out shopping because of too much stimulation.

For some children, being unable to communicate what they want is very frustrating. Sometimes, they try to communicate through body language and behavior such as crying, screaming, or arching their body toward something they want or away from something they do not want. In this case, tell your child that you understand that he is trying to tell you something. Offer him the thing that is likely to be what he wants such as a drink or a toy. It is useful to bring two or more possible objects and help him make a choice. Refer to Key 42 for communication suggestions.

Some children with cerebral palsy exhibit negative behavior because they are frustrated with failure. It can be overwhelming to be the only child who cannot hit a baseball or play tag. Comfort the child and help adapt the activity so he can participate and have fun. If behavior problems continue, remove the child from the frustrating situation. Changing the environment to be quieter and more rewarding is very helpful.

When you are working on problem behaviors, it is important to identify what behaviors are under your child's control and what behaviors are not realistic to expect him to control at this time. For example, hitting another child is often a behavior your child can voluntarily control. Wetting his pants may not be something that he can control at this time. Target behaviors your child is capable of controlling and then address them one at a time. Trust your instincts. Parents usually know. Once your child has mastered behaviors he can control, try behavioral management with other behaviors. He may now be able to stop wetting the bed or hitting himself.

Rewarding positive behaviors is much more effective than punishing negative behaviors. Use a very concrete reward that is meaningful for your child. Stickers on a chart, a token he can hold and count, a big hug, and lavish praise where you describe the specific behavior that pleased you are *very important*. Avoid giving your child food rewards or withholding favorite snacks. This can lead to obesity or problem eating behaviors. Avoid telling your child that he was *good* or *bad*. Instead say, "You did a terrific job helping to get dressed this morning," or "I liked it when you pushed your arm through the sleeve."

Both rewards and punishments should be immediate for most children with cerebral palsy. A long time between action and consequence will confuse any child. For some children, as time goes on, rewards can be spaced out for longer periods. For example, if the child can avoid having a temper tantrum for a whole school day, he can help the teacher pick up papers at the end of class or receive a sticker.

Withholding a privilege can be an effective way of disciplining any child. For a child with cerebral palsy who has a tantrum, turning off the television or music or taking away a favorite toy for a short period of time may work well. This approach gives the message that inappropriate behavior is a choice. A choice is something a child can control. Control feels good.

Making choices gives children some power. Tantrums and other problem behaviors are typically the result of a child feeling overwhelmed and out of control. Whenever possible, offer your child a choice. Take the extra time to work with switches, eye pointing, a communication board, or other devices to make your child's choices clear and understandable. When you offer your child a choice, always follow through with that choice and make sure that you find the options acceptable. Never offer a child a choice you cannot grant. Do not encourage your child to change his mind. If in the beginning you cannot understand your child's choice, slowly ask him to show you what he wants one more time. Next, use your words to frame your child's choice. "It looks like you chose to play with your car." Then, give your child the car.

Children with disabilities commonly try to manipulate people or expect special privileges because of their condition. Some children with cerebral palsy learn to encourage people to feel sorry for them or give them unfair advantages in social situations. Pity is often more disabling to a child than cerebral palsy itself. The family unit is the testing ground where children learn to behave and to develop a self-image. Pity should not be tolerated in your home and should be discouraged in the community because it further disables your child.

The best course of action is to make your home an empowerment home. Do not allow pity, sarcasm, name-calling, ridicule, or physical punishment. Do not allow your child to use his disability to gain unfair advantage over siblings or friends. An empowerment home is one where choice is encouraged and behavior has a predictable consequence. This strategy will help your child to function better in the real world.

Some children with cerebral palsy have behavior problems that may benefit from medication. In some cases of hyperactivity, short attention span, aggression, or self-injurious behavior, medication can be very helpful. The goal of behavioral medication is to balance a child's natural brain chemistry. Consult with your child's doctor to explore this option further.

Whatever plan you choose to help encourage and discipline your child, make sure that the same approach is used consistently at home, school, day care, church, and grandmother's house. If your child's behavior problems are very troublesome, a psychologist may be needed to evaluate your child and help you design a behavioral plan. A log recording your child's behavioral plan can be kept in the care notebook for all caregivers to follow. A loving and consistent approach to behavior and discipline should help your child with cerebral palsy learn the appropriate behaviors that will lead to a happier, more fulfilling life.

# PART SIX

## YOUR CHILD'S LEARNING

Children with disabilities need continuous opportunities to learn. Part Six discusses programs designed for infants and toddlers. Regular and special education programs as well as formal, written training plans are described. Part Six introduces you to the laws governing these programs and your rights as parents. It also gives strategies for helping your child with learning and communication. Using assistive technology or equipment for more independence is also reviewed. Especially look at Key 48 when reading Part Six, because transition planning is extremely important in the early intervention and school years.

# 33

# YOUR CHILD'S RIGHT TO EDUCATION: IT'S THE LAW

Before 1966 if children with disabilities received an education, it was provided at home or in state schools or institutions. In 1966, the *Elementary and Secondary Education Act Amendments* became the first federal law to make local public school systems responsible for educating children with disabilities. The *Education for All Handicapped Children Act* (EHA) of 1975 had a significant impact on education. This law entitled all children with disabilities to a *free appropriate public education*. Basically, this means that children, regardless of disability, can attend public school free of charge like other children.

Children are also entitled to education in the *least restrictive environment*. This means that as much as possible, a child who has a disability receives his schooling in settings with other children of the same age who do not have disabilities. Neighborhood schools are preferred. The least restrictive environment may differ for every child with a disability. One child may participate in regular classes independently or with an assistant. Another child may stay in a special education classroom with only children who have disabilities. An educational environment structured around lessening the restrictions on a child with disabilities provides a wide range of educational opportunities for that child.

In addition to providing for least restrictive environments, EHA ensured that services necessary for a child to benefit from education be provided by schools. These *related services* may include buses with wheelchair lifts, classroom aides, supplies, counseling, and therapy. Therapy provided in school must be directed toward helping a child to learn and participate in school activities. Examples include assisting a child with writing while she sits at a desk or teaching a child to propel a wheelchair through the busy cafeteria. Nursing or school health may be provided as a related service, also. For instance, a nurse may train teachers to suction or catheterize a student so that she can attend school all day.

Special education training plans were also initiated under EHA. Individualized education programs (IEPs) are written goals and teaching plans developed by an educational team for each child with a disability. The team includes teachers, parents, the student, and anyone else involved in the child's education, such as related service providers. IEPs will be discussed in more detail in Key 38.

The next legislative act to address the educational needs of children with disabilities, the *EHA Amendments*, was enacted in 1986. These amendments began the development of preschool programs for children with disabilities. Early intervention programs were also established by these 1986 amendments. Through these programs, infants and toddlers are provided with important early services. These programs were the first to focus on the family as well as the child. Individualized family service plans (IFSPs), similar to IEPs, are developed in early intervention. IFSPs are also discussed in Key 38. Early intervention is discussed in more detail in Key 36.

In 1990, the *Education for All Handicapped Children Act* was revised under new amendments and became the *Individuals with Disabilities Education Act* (IDEA). In addition to updating definitions, this law included transition planning and assistive technology in education plans for students with disabilities.

Table 3 addresses these laws and others that have had a tremendous impact on the lives of children and adults with disabilities. Undoubtedly, your child's rights have been improved by these laws. Revisions, new laws, developments in education, and society's views of people with disabilities will continue to influence your child's education.

**Table 3 MAJOR EDUCATION AND DISABILITY LAWS**

| Name | Law | Year | Main Issues |
|---|---|---|---|
| Elementary and Secondary Education Act Amendments | PL-89-750 | 1966 | Provided federal government grant money for education at local school level instead of in state institutions. |
| Rehabilitation Act, Section 504 | PL-93-112 | 1973 | Required equal rights, accessibility, and rehabilitation services, regardless of severity of disability, in federally funded programs like schools. |
| Education for All Handicapped Children Act (EHA) | PL-94-142 | 1975 | Free appropriate public education. Least restrictive environment. Related Services. IEPs. Ages 5 through 21 years. |
| EHA Amendments | PL-99-457 | 1986 | Preschool programs. Ages 3 to 5 years. Part H set up early intervention programs and IFSPs. Ages 0 to 3 years. |
| Carl D. Perkins Vocational and Applied Technology Education Act | PL-101-392 | 1990 | Vocational education programs—job training and placement. |
| Individuals with Disabilities Education Act (IDEA) | PL-101-476 | 1990 | Renamed and expanded EHA. Transition planning and assistive technology added to IEP. |
| Americans with Disabilities Act | PL-101-336 | 1990 | Guarantees full civil rights of all people with disabilities. Major influence on day cares, restaurants, workplaces, and other settings. |
| IDEA Amendments | PL-102-119 | 1991 | Set up Federal Interagency Coordinating Council. Stressed early intervention and professional development. |
| Rehabilitation Act Amendments | PL-102-569 | 1992 | High school level transition planning must include rehabilitation and assistive technology services. |

Sources: Adapted from Jeanne L. Fischer, "Physical Therapy in Educational Environments," *Pediatric Physical Therapy* Vol. 6, no. 3 (1994): 144–147; and Lizanne DeStefano and Dale T. Snauwaert, *A Value-Critical Approach to Transition Policy Analysis*. (Champaign, IL: University of Illinois, Secondary Transition Intervention Effectiveness Institute, 1989). Laura F. Rothstein, *Special Education Law* (White Plains, NY: Longman, 1990).

# 34

# YOUR RIGHTS AS A PARENT

Federal education laws require that school systems include parents in the education of their children with disabilities. Parents have the right and responsibility to be an active participant in their child's learning from before to beyond the school years. You have an important role to play in making sure that your child receives the best education and services possible. Your rights as a parent, specifically as they apply to education, will be discussed here.

**Right to Consent**

Your written approval is necessary before your child can be evaluated for services like early intervention or special education. Before any tests can be performed, on a child's hearing or intelligence for example, a parent must consent to the testing. Parents must also give consent for their child to begin educational programs. Your signature on your child's written training plan indicates that you agree with your child's placement and program.

**Right to Participation**

As previously discussed, education laws clearly state that parents have the right to participate actively in planning and designing their child's learning programs. In addition to having an important role in developing individualized family service plans (IFSPs) during early intervention programs, parents are also identified as individualized education program (IEP) team members during the school years.

## YOUR RIGHTS AS A PARENT

Parents are to be notified of all IEP and follow-up meetings. The school must allow parents to agree to a time and date before scheduling meetings. If you need an interpreter or wish to have an advocate attend, this can be arranged. If you cannot attend the meeting in person, the school must allow you to participate in another way, such as through telephone calls, letters, or other forms of communication.

During meetings, parents and school personnel discuss the child's educational and service needs, and decide on goals, programs, and services to be delivered. The meeting is an ideal time for you to become fully informed about your child's education and to discuss your expectations for your child and the program. Additionally, you should discuss the needs of your family and its ability to follow through with training at home.

Keep in mind that you are an equal partner in your child's learning. Your participation provides consistency from year to year. You know your child better than anyone else does.

### Right to Challenge Decisions

If you disagree with a recommendation made by your child's school, you have a right to voice your opinions and concerns. For example, you may feel that your child needs to be placed in another class. If the school does not agree with you, you should both come to a compromise. Your child could have a trial period in the desired class with an ongoing assessment of his progress. After the trial period, a final decision will be made based on how well he did in the class. You also have the right to request an independent evaluation of your child if you disagree with the results of a particular professional's assessment of your child's abilities.

You and your child's other IEP members should be able to find solutions and make compromises as a team. You can request another IEP meeting to discuss the issues further. The school district may choose to have a third party provide *mediation*. This unbiased person or group will listen to both sides of the issues and recommend a course of action. Mediation is used for coming to a peaceful solution.

Even after mediation, parents still have the right to file a formal complaint and receive a state-level review of the situation. A legal process was developed through special education laws that allows parents to appeal decisions made by school districts. *Due process*, as this formal procedure is called, involves meetings between parents, school representatives, and a state-appointed impartial hearing officer. As with mediation, the officer makes a recommendation after hearing statements from parents and the school. If you disagree with the results of the due process hearing, you can seek legal action and take the school district to court.

**Right to Privacy**

As a parent, you have a right to review the records kept by the school on your child. The records include reports on evaluations, health, performance, and behavior and letters to you. You should keep copies of your child's IEPs and other appropriate records because the school district will only keep them for a certain number of years. You can request that inaccurate records be changed. You can also ask school personnel to explain the records to you.

Contact your state Department of Education for more information on your rights as a parent of a child with a disability. It can also give you the guidelines for filing an appeal. The state Department of Education or the National Information Center for Children and Youth with Disabilities (NICHCY) can provide you with the most current information on state and federal education legislation. Parent Training and Information (PTI) Centers in each state provide individual and group training on parents' rights and other important issues. Contact NICHCY and Technical Assistance for Parent Programs (TAPP) to learn about your local PTI and much more. These and other resources can be found at the back of this book. By understanding your rights, you can improve your child's education and overall experience in school.

# 35

# COMPREHENSIVE EVALUATIONS

Children at risk for disabilities receive many types of evaluations. Your child has probably already undergone many evaluations for medical and diagnostic reasons. More evaluations are necessary, though, before your son or daughter can receive special services such as those provided by health departments or schools. In fact, a comprehensive multidisciplinary evaluation is needed to qualify your child for early intervention programs. Early intervention, a program paid for by the government, is discussed in detail in Key 36.

*Comprehensive* means that everything about your child will be evaluated. Sometimes, one person does the comprehensive evaluation, but most of the time, evaluations will be *multidisciplinary*. This means that people from various disciplines or professions such as occupational therapy, nursing, speech pathology, and psychology will look at and test your child. Each person will evaluate different areas of your child's development. They may perform segments of the evaluation separately. If a team approach is used, the terms *interdisciplinary* or *transdisciplinary* describe the style of teamwork. The multiple disciplines represented by this combined group of professionals provide a comprehensive or detailed assessment of your child's abilities.

Your participation as a parent or guardian is very important. Often, your observations of your child are the main source of information for the evaluators. They rely on your reports especially if your child is being uncooperative because of the test environment.

Most evaluators understand that children do better in a natural setting like their home instead of being in a clinic.

An overall evaluation of your child is performed to see if there are areas of developmental delay. Your child's ability to perform developmental skills or *milestones* is compared with the time periods when children without disabilities achieve the milestones. For example, at eighteen months old, a typical child will walk upstairs with help, match sounds to animals, and play by herself for a few minutes at a time. If your child is not performing a skill at the expected time, your child may have a developmental delay. Standardized formal tests are used to compare typical children and those who are developing more slowly. Many types of tests are available for evaluations.

Your child's performance on the evaluation will determine whether or not she qualifies for services. Delayed development of a certain percentage or amount in one or more of the following areas qualifies a child for early intervention: physical, cognitive, language, speech, psychosocial, or self-help skills. Because children with cerebral palsy have a high risk of being developmentally delayed, a diagnosis of cerebral palsy will generally qualify the child for services. In that case, the comprehensive evaluation serves as a baseline, and your child's future progress can be compared with it.

Infant evaluations include examining reflexes and observing how your baby performs specific developmental skills like looking at objects, holding her head up, rolling, sitting, playing, crawling, and so on. It also includes areas such as your child's swallowing, nutrition, temperament, response to touch and sounds, mental abilities or cognition, and early speech skills.

Toddlers and older children receive similar evaluations. Their performance is compared with children of their same age who do not have disabilities. A comprehensive assessment is performed to qualify your child for services provided by schools, such as special education. As your child grows older, further evaluations may be necessary so that she can take part in other services like regular education or job training. Another example of a formal evaluation your child may eventually take is a college entrance exam.

# 36

# WHAT IS EARLY INTERVENTION?

The federal government created Public Law 99-457, part H, of the *Education of the Handicapped Act Amendments of 1986* requiring states to provide programs for infants and toddlers at risk for or diagnosed with disabilities. These services are called *early intervention* or, in some states, *early childhood intervention*. Children between the ages of zero and three years are served by these programs. Funding for early intervention is provided by state and federal governments. Your child can participate free of charge.

Early intervention consists of health, social, and educational services for both the child and family. The *family unit* is the focus of early intervention. It is hard enough for a family to learn that a child has special needs, much less deal with the complex issues involved in raising this child alone. Therefore, early intervention programs exist to assist you in as many ways as possible. A goal of early intervention is to help families become competent and independent at caring for a child with a disability.

Involving parents in the early stimulation of a child, particularly one who is delayed, benefits the child. When a family actively participates in early intervention, the child will grow to have greater potential. By working with a young child early, some of the problems associated with cerebral palsy can be reduced. The child can then be more independent as he grows older.

As mentioned in the previous Key, a comprehensive evaluation is completed before a child enters an early intervention program.

After the evaluation and notifying you of your son's or daughter's qualification process, a meeting is set up with the family and various professionals. During the meeting, you develop a plan for your child called the *individualized family services plan* (IFSP). The IFSP document will be discussed in detail in Key 38. In the IFSP meeting, held every six to twelve months, parents and chosen professionals discuss the child's and the family's strengths and needs. You identify your goals and areas where you need or want some guidance. From this plan, specific services and team members are determined. Your child's IFSP team may consist of only a few members: child, parents, case manager, and primary service provider. The team may also consist of additional professionals who may serve as direct service providers, consultants, or advisors. After the IFSP meeting, you will have a game plan and teammates.

The case manager can be a great asset to your family. This person can educate you about your child's diagnosis, local support groups, community resources, and much more. The case manager can help to coordinate all of the services your child receives.

In early intervention programs, using a *transdisciplinary* team model, a primary service provider is designated by the IFSP team based on your child's or your family's immediate needs. The following are some examples. If your child has uncontrolled seizures, substantial breathing problems, or is otherwise medically fragile, a nurse might initially be the primary service provider. An occupational therapist may be chosen if your child has swallowing or eating problems, or has poor use of his hands. A physical therapist may be designated if your main concern is the way your child moves. If your child's behavior or your family's ability to cope with the stress of having a child with disabilities must be addressed immediately, a psychologist is named as the primary service provider. Additionally, an older child in early intervention may need more emphasis on speech skills and, therefore, a speech language pathologist would lead the team.

Of course, you and your child may need all of these services in the first three years. As mentioned, the primary service provider specializes in the most immediate area of need. Other areas are not neglected, though. In early intervention programs, service providers receive general training in the skills of other disciplines. For instance, the nurse working with a more medically involved child may teach parents positioning and exercises as well as medical procedures. The physical therapist may encourage communication skills while helping an infant learn to sit. A speech pathologist, while enhancing speech, may also monitor swallowing and support the family emotionally. The primary service provider should call on consultants from other disciplines for ideas and family training. Also, the primary service provider may change as the family's or child's needs change.

By using primary service providers, early intervention programs make things a little easier on you. You and your child do not have to bond with more than one person at a time. You are not subjected to the same questions from many different people. You have only one person giving you suggestions and training. You do not have as many appointments to keep or more than one person coming to your home.

However, each community's early intervention program is different. A primary service provider may not be used in some areas. Instead, your family may have several people providing services to you at one time. This *interdisciplinary* type of team model can have benefits. Sometimes more than one professional is necessary to address your child's complex needs.

The location of early intervention services varies. Ideally, services are provided in the most natural environment for your child, usually your home. Your child will respond better and more consistently in a familiar, comfortable setting. Usually, the service provider will come to your home the number of times per week or month determined as necessary by the IFSP team. Intervention is often received in center-based programs once a child is two years old. Sometimes, services are provided in a day care or preschool setting if this is where your child spends his time. Infrequently, an infant is seen in a clinical setting like a hospital's outpatient therapy department or at a public health center.

Through home-based therapy and primary service providers, early intervention establishes a basis for family-centered service. As indicated, the family is the focus in early intervention. A very important service is family training. The professionals will give the parents, siblings, grandparents, and other care providers as much knowledge and skill as possible so that the family can care for the child in the best possible manner. The therapists teach you how to give the special care your baby needs. More frequent visits will be needed at first as you learn how to help your child do as much as he can. As you become more independent and can handle caring for and teaching your child on your own, the service provider will come less often. If the family and child show a need for more services, the frequency of services will increase again. Examples would be if your child's health changed or if he started to learn a new skill, like walking, that required more training from a therapist.

When your child is two years old, the IFSP team must develop a transition plan for the next stage of life. This plan will help to coordinate services between early intervention and the public schools, which are responsible for children with disabilities ages three to twenty-one. Refer to Key 48 for more information on transition planning.

Whether or not your child qualifies for early intervention, be sure to expose him to as much therapy and education as possible at an early age. Stimulate your infant and toddler in all areas of development. Investigate good preschool options as well. Your child's future depends on an early start.

# 37

# REGULAR AND SPECIAL EDUCATION

Most people participated in *regular education* programs in school, even if they attended a private school. They had regular teachers in typical classrooms with the usual types of classwork. Maybe they knew kids in special education or LD (learning disability) classes. A child who used a wheelchair or walked differently might have been at their school. More than likely they never had children with cerebral palsy in their classes.

This image is what most people think of when they think of school. On the other hand, most people may think of *special education* as what goes on in the classrooms at the end of the hall or in the portable buildings behind the school, where the "kids with disabilities or retardation go." Special education, in recent years, has developed into so much more.

Special education is a set of services determined by law through the *Individuals with Disabilities Education Act* (IDEA). It is designed to meet the educational needs of all children with disabilities. Special education services can include many things such as methods of instruction, class placement, related services, an individualized education program (IEP), and a special education teacher.

A special education teacher has a college degree and, in most states, a master's degree. The focus of special education training programs is different from those for regular education teachers. Classes for special education teachers include learning about cerebral palsy, learning disabilities, mental retardation, and emotional and behavioral disturbances. Strategies to help children learn are taught and practiced. To complete their training, several months of student teaching is performed under the direction of an experienced special education teacher. A special education teacher may evaluate your child, teach her in different settings, or consult with her other school teachers.

A comprehensive evaluation can be performed at your child's school to determine if she needs special instruction or teaching methods to learn. This evaluation will qualify her to receive special education services. An IEP meeting will then be held in order to identify team members and necessary services. You and the rest of the team may decide that your child would benefit the most by placement in a class with other children who have special needs and by having a specially trained teacher. Your child's class placement will depend on her age. In this case, the word placement means class assignment and not the location of the classroom.

Your child may not always need to be in a special education class for the full day. She may improve in her learning skills to where she can attend regular education classes part or all of the school day. *Resource room* instruction may be all that your child needs in order to benefit from her regular education program. A resource room is where a special education teacher can review lessons and assignments. Using appropriate methods, the special education teacher and student work on the student's skills that need improvement. Instead of a resource room, your child may need only *consultation* from a special education teacher in order to attend regular education classes. A special education teacher would talk with you and your child's regular education teacher or teachers as often as needed to make suggestions, give advice, and help to solve problems.

The degree to which your child participates in special education depends on her needs, your expectations and goals, and the team members' level of training, experience, and creativity. Key 40 will give you more information about including students who have cerebral palsy in classes with students who do not have disabilities. *Mainstreaming* or *inclusion* are the terms used to describe this topic. Also refer to Key 48 about transition, which covers the importance of planning for changes in your child's educational placement.

Related services are provided to enhance your child's learning and to make certain she can attend school. Therapy, transportation, ramps, elevators, and communication devices are a few examples. These services would be listed in your child's IEP if she is served through special education.

If your child with cerebral palsy is in regular education and does not receive any of the various special education services, her rights are protected by the *Rehabilitation Act*. Section 504 of this law provides services to assist your child so that she can participate in school. It also covers adaptations to the school environment. It could include any of the related services or supports mentioned above and more. The specific adaptations would be written in your child's 504 Plan. The difference with this plan is that the services are not needed for academic reasons as they are in special education; they are needed solely for your child's *equal participation* in a regular education program. The services allow your child to participate in school just like any other child.

It is possible that your child with cerebral palsy has the intelligence and the physical abilities to attend school without any assistance or adaptations. As she grows older, keep in mind the services and laws mentioned in this Key. They might be needed at a later time. Your child may change schools and want to participate in programs like drivers' education or sports, or her abilities or goals may change over time.

# 38

# TRAINING PLANS: IFSP, IEP, AND IHP

This Key discusses three types of training plans: the individualized family services plan (IFSP), the individualized education program (IEP), and the individualized habilitation plan (IHP).

**Individualized Family Services Plan—IFSP**

An IFSP document is written every six to twelve months when a child is in early intervention. It is reviewed and revised as needed. The IFSP is developed by parents and professionals through teamwork. After your child and his development have been evaluated, the family's strengths and needs are also identified. During the IFSP meeting, the team discusses ways to meet the needs of the child and the family and how to build on your strengths.

Your child's development and your family are the focus of the IFSP. With this in mind, general goals are written for the above-mentioned needs. Goals may also be called outcomes, meaning *what you expect the training to accomplish*. For example, an infant named Joe has the following needs: eating better, family education, and financial assistance. Goal 1: Joe will finish a bottle in a reasonable amount of time. Goal 2: Joe's parents will learn positioning and feeding techniques. Goal 3: Joe's family will contact resources from a list provided by the case manager. Two-year-old Ashley, on the other hand, will have the following goals for meeting her needs of exploring her environment and communicating her desires. Goal 1: Ashley will move by herself to get a toy. Goal 2: Ashley will point to or say the name of something she wants. Goal 3: Ashley's parents will learn ways to encourage Ashley to do more by herself. Strategies are then designed to meet goals.

Strategies tell you what steps will be taken over the next six to twelve months to teach your child new skills. In this way, the IFSP serves as a written game plan for achieving the goals within a specific time frame.

During the IFSP meeting, you decide on what services you and your family will receive as well as how and when they will be provided. Options for services could include therapy, location, counseling, transportation, equipment, and health. Team members will give their opinions, and the family will make the ultimate decision. Finally, a transition plan is written into the IFSP to prepare the child for his next step in life, school.

**Individualized Education Program—IEP**

If your child with cerebral palsy enters special education, an IEP is written to direct his school program. Although the family continues to be very important, the student and his education are the focus of the training plan or IEP. Your child's team now includes a special education teacher. Sometimes, a regular education teacher is also on the team, depending on your child's abilities. School administrators may also serve as team members.

At the beginning of each school year, the child, parents, and IEP team meet to determine needs, strengths, and annual goals. In addition, short-term objectives or small goals are written as steps toward achieving major annual goals. The IEP also outlines how progress on these goals will be measured or what criteria must be met for the child to have reached the objectives and goals. The IEP of a student who is learning to spell and use a computer might include the following. Goal: Juan will complete a spelling assignment on the class computer by the end of the year. Objective 1: Through the use of adapted switches and seating, Juan will correctly match first letters of words to their pictures by the end of the first nine weeks. Objective 2: With the above equipment, Juan will spell five words with picture cues by the end of the semester. Further objectives will build toward the annual goal.

As you can see, IEP goals are more specific than those on an IFSP. Goals must be appropriate for the child's age, meaningful, and educational. A creative team can make goals and strategies that will work for your child. It might take a lot of effort, but school can be a learning environment even for a child with the most severe disabilities. Children with severe physical disabilities or mental retardation may work on very simple goals throughout the school years, depending on their functioning level. However, their goals must still be *meaningful*.

The IEP team will also determine and document the related services that are necessary for your child to attend and fully participate in school. Related services include nursing, adapted physical education, supplies, modified meals, accessible buildings, a classroom aide, and so on. The school is responsible for making sure that your son or daughter can go to each class and other areas of the school. If necessary, ramps will be built and bathrooms will be modified. An aide can be assigned to assist your child at school. As necessary, the aide will accompany the child to class, help to complete classwork, write on the blackboard, and feed and change him. The aide's tasks are as varied as your child's abilities.

Physical and occupational therapy, speech language pathology, audiology, vocational training, and vision training are also related services. Therapists who work in schools are responsible for helping children with disabilities to perform better at school. These services must be related to education. For example, instead of the more traditional form of physical therapy where students were taken to the therapy room for stretching or walking exercises, therapists now must make therapy part of learning. Exercises are performed in physical education. A student will work on how well he walks in the classroom or in the hall on the way to the cafeteria.

During the IEP meeting, the team determines how, when, and to what extent these services will occur. Therapists may initially work directly with the child and instruct the teacher and aides in therapy skills. The therapist may then pull away and provide consultation or advise as needed. If direct therapy is needed later, it can be added again with an IEP review meeting.

Like an IFSP, the IEP should include a transition plan. In school, a child is always transitioning or moving into a different class, setting, or grade. A transition plan will help your son or daughter adjust to these changes better. Transition planning is discussed in Key 48.

## Individualized Habilitation Plan—IHP

If your child receives services through the Department of Human Services or other agencies, an individualized habilitation plan may be necessary. IHPs are most often used in residential settings like group homes or state institutions. They may also be used if an aide or habilitation training specialist provides home services.

In either case, an IHP document is much like an IFSP or IEP. An IHP meeting is held where team members determine needs, write goals, establish services, and plan for the future. The IHP is different in that goals are not just related to development or education. *Habilitation* means learning a skill. The IHP is structured around what your child knows and what he needs to learn to be more independent.

The IHP may focus on certain areas like self-care, vocational or job training, community management or getting around in your hometown, recreation, and communication. An example of a goal for a younger child with cerebral palsy would be that Emily will use a spoon with hand-over-hand assistance to eat 75 percent of her meal. A teenager's goal might be that after receiving his paycheck from work, Travis will take public transportation to deposit it in the bank three months in a row.

The IHP will include all aspects of training and should be on target with your child's IEP if he is still in school. After graduation, an IHP may be your child's only training plan. If he is in a specific job-training program, he may have a plan similar to an IHP.

In conclusion, various training plans or programs are written for children and adults with disabilities. They serve as a road map for your child's expected progress. You should keep copies of the plans because the agency or school will not keep them for very many years.

# 39

# WORKING WITH YOUR CHILD'S EDUCATION TEAM

A child's education team consists of the child, her parents, teachers, related service providers, a case manager, and, possibly, school system personnel who monitor the process. The roles of each team member have been discussed in the previous Keys. Throughout this book teamwork between parents and professionals has been stressed.

You, your family, your child, her teacher, and her service providers are partners. You can accomplish a lot if you work together. Know the name and phone number of service providers. This seems like such a simple thing, but parents frequently do not know the name of their child's school therapist. Ideally, they would have met at an individualized education program (IEP) meeting or, at least, the therapist and parents would have talked on the phone. Sometimes, however, this does not happen. You can make sure that you are working as partners by contacting the professionals yourself.

Do not let the professionals "run you over" in IEP meetings. They may just report to you and tell you their plan for your child. The meetings are meant to allow planning and discussion as an entire team. You are all supposed to come up with a plan together.

Do not limit communication about your child to specific meeting times. Let the service providers know what your child is doing at home and how you would like her to improve. Ask how things are going in the classroom, in therapy, or in job training. Ask for progress reports at frequent intervals like every week or month if they are not already being provided. Visit your child at school, day care, therapy, or her home if she does not live with you. Meet with the professionals with and without your child present.

Before, during, and after the school years, let the professionals who work with your child know what you expect of them. Most professionals have training in working with parents, but they sometimes need reminders. Let them know when something is not clear to you. Repeat what someone has said in your own words. Keep notes for yourself, especially when you exchange information outside of a meeting.

If you want information on your child's condition, parent support groups, resources, funding, respite, home care, transportation, or anything else, let your team members know. Ask about other services for your child and how to get in touch with them. Share the information or resources you have gathered. If either you or the professionals hit a road block, work on a solution together. Ask for help from other service providers or parents.

The best way for parents and professionals to work together is to listen to each other. You also need a common vision of your child's potential. Let them know that it is okay to disagree with you, but you still expect their support. If you disagree with them, be polite. Find out if you are just misunderstanding each other. Come to a compromise when possible. Once you understand what to expect from each other, you can work as a team to help your child live life to its fullest.

# 40

# WHAT ARE MAINSTREAMING AND INCLUSION?

Some children with cerebral palsy go to special schools only for children with disabilities. Others attend public schools, but remain in their special education classroom all day and do not interact with children without disabilities. Still other children with cerebral palsy attend regular education classes and are fully involved with other children their own age.

Schooling for children with cerebral palsy of all ages falls along a continuous scale from the most separated and isolated to the most included and involved. The first example above shows how a child with a disability can be removed entirely from the community and placed in a special school where he is separated from children without disabilities. These schools can be very educational, but they do isolate children from the rest of the community.

The second example is fairly typical of American schools. The amount of separation can vary from school to school. At some schools, children in the special education classes will attend schoolwide events like assemblies or eat in the cafeteria. At others, they will share certain classes, like art or music, with children who are not disabled. As the scale continues toward the third example above, the child with cerebral palsy becomes more and more included in regular education.

*Mainstreaming* is a word used in the education world to describe the participation in regular education of a child or children

## WHAT ARE MAINSTREAMING AND INCLUSION?

with disabilities. Educators say that the child is in the mainstream just like other children. Traditionally, only people with mild mental retardation or mild physical disabilities have been mainstreamed.

Over the past several years, children with more complex mental, physical, or medical disabilities have been included in regular education classes. The extent or level of *inclusion* varies. Special educators seem to use the word inclusion more today than the word mainstreaming.

Inclusion is an ideal in the education world. Inclusion takes into account educating *all* children and adolescents in age-appropriate, regular education classes at schools within their neighborhoods. It also involves supporting the teachers and students so that inclusion is successful. Special education teachers are trained to be consultants to other teachers. They help develop IEPs for students and provide continuous advice on educating and handling children with disabilities. Therapists, adapted physical education teachers, and other service providers also support inclusion through direct, integrated, and consultation services.

The easiest time to include your child in education settings with nondisabled peers may be in regular day care, preschool, and kindergarten programs. At this age, children are just learning about other children and your child's differences might not seem so different. Elementary school is the most important time for full inclusion because the students are learning basic education as well as rules, verbal skills, and social skills. In higher elementary school, students with and without disabilities can do schoolwork side by side or in groups. They can help each other learn.

If your child has been included in regular education in primary school, the transition to secondary education should not be too difficult. Inclusion in junior high, middle school, and high school, as in earlier grades, can be total or class specific. Your child may attend regular social studies classes and special language arts or math classes. As your child grows older, keep his goals in mind. If he is totally included in regular education classes, make sure that he is getting the life skills training he may need in the future. For instance, special education classes for teenagers must help the students gain skills for work and independent living. Talk with your child's team about life skills training opportunities at school and home. For information on transition and vocational training, refer to Keys 48 and 49.

Why is it important for children with cerebral palsy to be around other children who are not disabled? The other children can be role models or examples for your child. Playing with and sitting by a peer can motivate your child to try things that are difficult for him. Inclusion also gives your child a much wider range of learning opportunities than has ever been available before to children with cerebral palsy. It can help him to improve many of his skills. Inclusion also provides children in regular education with a friend and example of someone who has a disability. This can do a lot for reducing prejudice in the world. You might choose against inclusion, however. You may feel that it will frustrate your child, hinder learning, or put him at risk for injuries or rejection. Of course, these things can happen in special education classes or to children without disabilities as well.

Deciding if inclusion or mainstreaming is right for your child is a personal choice. Remember that the amount of inclusion can vary for each child and over periods of time. How well your child does with inclusion or in regular classes does not depend on him as much as it does on the commitment, creativity, and positive attitude of his teachers, school administrators, and family.

# 41

# HELPING YOUR CHILD LEARN

Have you ever thought about how you learn? Do you learn new information better when you hear it, see it, or feel it? Do you need to repeat or talk through the information out loud or do you need time to think about it on your own and let the information sink in? If you are learning something new, do you like to watch someone else do it first and then try it? How many times do you need to practice the skill before you are good at it?

People learn in different ways. Teachers use particular learning methods with each child so that every student has an opportunity to learn the best way she can. The student's intelligence, experience, interests, and ability to see, hear, and move help the teacher determine the child's own learning style. This is important whether you are teaching algebra, history, putting on a shirt, driving, sitting up, playing baseball, or the alphabet. Ask your child's teacher what works best, and try to use the same style at home.

Many people with cerebral palsy learn more slowly and need more practice than other people. Skills that involve movement usually require a lot of training time. Give your son or daughter a chance to try a movement skill, like getting up from the floor or playing with a toy. Tell your child how to do the skill. Gradually give more help if needed.

You can use your hands to guide your child through the movement, but give only as much assistance as necessary. You might need to move her through every part of the movement at first. It is hoped that, over time, the amount of help she needs from you will decrease, and she will be able to do part or all of the movement by herself. For example, you can help your child draw by holding a crayon in her hand and guiding her hand on the paper. As she learns to move the crayon, give less guidance until she is drawing by herself. Sometimes, your child will need a piece of equipment, such as a special pencil holder, spoon, or chair, to help her perform movement skills. Her therapists can help with making or ordering adaptive equipment or by changing the skill so she can learn it more easily.

A good way to help your child learn is to make it easier for her to concentrate on what she is learning. Try to reduce the number of things that can distract her, like the television or interruptions from her siblings. In this way, your child can pay attention to what she is doing.

Because your child may respond more slowly when you ask her to do something, give her more time. Let her think about the instructions. *Pause* before you repeat the instructions. If she does not start to act after you have waited a little while, demonstrate the activity for her. It is especially important to show your child how to do skills that are new to her. Most people learn by watching others.

Sometimes, your child might need you to show her how to do something even if she has done it before. This can be a reminder and help her to start an activity. Often, the best teachers are the child's brothers and sisters. All children learn from each other. Being role models is another good way to involve siblings and make them feel important.

When you teach your child, instruct using short sentences. You may not be able to give her multiple steps to follow like, "Go down the street and turn left." You may need to break down a skill into simple parts and give her time to do each part one by one. Toothbrushing is a good example. "Take the cap off of the tube of toothpaste." "Put toothpaste on your toothbrush." "Brush your teeth." "Get a drink." "Rinse off your brush." "Replace the cap." Your child may or may not need such simple instructions.

Encourage your child when she is doing something correctly. Letting her know that she is doing well and that you are proud of her will make her feel good about herself. It will make her want to do better each time. You can also give your child information about how and why she did something correctly. "I like the way you held up your head when you answered me." "It worked better because you closed your mouth on the spoon this time." These types of comments give your child more information than simply saying, "That was better." You can also tell her how to make improvements by saying something like, "Try it again, but next time do it this way and see what happens." Descriptive instructions are much more helpful than telling your child she is wrong or that she cannot do something.

Children with cerebral palsy, like other children, need opportunities to discover things on their own. This includes letting them make some mistakes. It is important for children to learn through trial and error, with positive remarks and encouragement from their parents. In this way, your child will learn what works and what does not. Her sense of accomplishment will be worth any minor frustration she might feel during the effort.

These are only a few tips about your child's learning. Every child, skill, and situation is different. If something does not work, try it another way. Ask your child's teachers and therapists for suggestions. In some cases, asking your child for ideas can be helpful, too. Get suggestions from other parents. Be patient with your child and yourself because every child is capable of learning.

# 42

# HELPING YOUR CHILD COMMUNICATE

Communicating with each other is one of the most important things people do. Without a means of communication, people cannot exchange information and ideas, express emotions, or ask for help. Giving your child a way to do these things will improve her independence and self-esteem. In addition to the strategies mentioned in Key 41, learning tips can help your child communicate.

Children with cerebral palsy usually need to be positioned well in order to communicate. Positioning to support the body will improve the quality of a child's speech. Her voice may be louder and easier to understand. Positioning will also improve her ability to use other body parts to communicate if she cannot speak. Good posture and support are necessary in all positions but are especially critical when your child is sitting. Ask your child's therapists for suggestions on how to position her to improve communication.

By talking to your child, you help her learn about communication. Tell your baby about things around her and what you are doing together. Talk when you change her diaper. Describe her toys. Point out the names of things in your home. Use simple and complex words and not just baby talk. Use the same methods as your child grows older, but continue to increase the complexity of your descriptions. Tell your child how things work and why. Talk to

## HELPING YOUR CHILD COMMUNICATE

your young, adolescent, or adult child with cerebral palsy as you would to any person of the same age. Talking and using age-appropriate language are very important even if you think that your child does not understand. You will not only be treating your child with respect but also exposing her to information and language.

Language is not only *expressive*, it is also *receptive*. People easily relate to the expressive side of communication. They talk, write, type, or use body language to send messages. Receptive language, or receiving messages, involves understanding the messages received and is more difficult to identify when happening. People gain information through all of their senses, not just hearing. In order to communicate effectively, people use their expressive and receptive language skills together.

Knowledge of how children typically learn to communicate may help you teach your child. Language skills usually develop after a child has mastered early mental and social skills. Cognitively, infants learn about their world. They begin to understand important things like *cause and effect*. Socially, infants learn to interact with the world. They cry, make faces, and gesture by moving their bodies. Young infants first learn how to make simple sounds. Next, they experiment with the sounds. Children then build on their developing social and mental skills. Gradually, their sounds become more complicated and meaningful until they are talking. These development issues are discussed in more detail in Keys 17, 19, and 20.

In order to talk, children must coordinate their mouth, jaw, voice box, and breathing pattern. This takes practice. Your child with cerebral palsy may work on language coordination skills with a speech language pathologist. This professional will use strategies to improve your child's voice quality and the way she says words. Attend therapy sessions and use the strategies at home to help your child learn to speak well.

If your child cannot talk, find other ways for her to communicate. One of the most simple ways to communicate is by answering yes/no questions. Find a body movement or expression that your child can consistently do on purpose. Head nods and shakes may be an option that can be understood by other people. If your child has poor control of her head, she might use smiles and frowns, eye blinks, or movements of her arms, hands, fingers, or legs. She might make noises that together you have decided mean yes or no. Let others know what your child's responses mean.

Your child needs a way to communicate beyond answering yes/no questions. Perhaps your child can use her hands well enough to learn sign language. Many children with cerebral palsy who cannot talk or who are difficult to understand use true and modified forms of sign language. Others learn to communicate using elaborate word symbols.

Many children with cerebral palsy who cannot speak use simple picture symbols to express themselves. Pictures that represent people, objects, and actions can be arranged to make *communication boards*. Your child could point to, move her hand on top of, or look at the desired picture. Someone else would interpret her action and make a response. For example, if the child looks at a picture of a cup, someone would get her a drink. The child would then be offered a choice of beverages, and she would answer yes or no. Ideally, the communication board would have choices on it like pictures of a carton of milk, a can of cola, and a glass of juice. Perhaps the child would point to the picture of a toilet. A parent could say to the child, "OK, I'll take you to the bathroom." Photographs of familiar objects, people, and activities can also be used for a communication board. Photographs are sometimes easier for a child to relate to because they are of real things instead of stick figures. Photographs and pictures can be made into books instead of mounted on boards or wheelchair trays. A child who walks can carry the communication book wherever she goes.

Communication boards, books, symbols, and sign language are examples of *alternative* forms of communication. Speech language pathologists are primarily responsible for determining the best form of communication for a person with a disability. *Augmentative and alternative communication* (AAC) devices are a type of assistive technology described in Key 43. Sophisticated types of AAC devices are generally electronic or battery operated.

AAC in any form can be tremendously beneficial to people who cannot talk.

You can help your child to be successful at using these communication options by helping the other team members make decisions. How will your child use the communication board or device? Where will it be placed in order for her to use it most effectively? What messages would your child like to say? When will she use it? Is she ready for something more complicated?

You should encourage your child to use her communication method always. Use the method at home. Have your child take her device back and forth to school. She cannot communicate if her "voice" is not available. Ask her questions in such a way that she would have to use the method in order to answer. Instead of a yes/no question that she could answer with a head nod, ask open-ended questions. "What would you like for lunch?" "What did you do at school?" It is also important to give your child sufficient time to answer you. *Pause* after you ask for a response. Give more prompts for her to communicate as needed. Pausing and prompting are good strategies for encouraging communication in children who use their voices as well as those who use AAC.

A very important way you can help your child communicate is by being quiet. Let her initiate conversation. Adults tend to dominate interactions with children who have disabilities. Adults need to give children a chance to start talking instead of always just answering questions. You can set up social situations where your child can communicate with her peers. A playground, Sunday school, or Grandpa's house are places where she might communicate with little guidance from an adult. When someone talks to your child, try very hard not to answer for her. Do not anticipate what she is going to say or put words in her mouth.

Teach your child to use the way she communicates appropriately. She should not continuously push the same button. Use behavior management strategies if she does. Hearing "I want some candy" over and over through your child's AAC might drive you crazy. It would be nice, though, if you had to ask your child with cerebral palsy, "Please be quiet."

# 43

# WHAT IS ASSISTIVE TECHNOLOGY?

All people use technology to make their lives easier, safer, and more productive. From the rubber jar opener used to remove the pickle lid, to the helmet construction workers wear, to the satellite that lets people watch events happening around the world, everyone is surrounded by technology.

*Assistive technology*, also called adaptive equipment, enables people with disabilities to participate in activities as independently as possible. More than likely, your child has used various types of assistive technology already. Assistive technology of a medical nature might include an incubator, a suction machine, a helmet to protect your child if he has seizures, a feeding tube, glasses, hearing aids, or ankle braces.

Therapists may recommend equipment that can help your child learn developmental skills. Walkers, therapy balls, positioning chairs, and handles on toys are examples. Your child may also need assistive technology for eating, dressing, going to the bathroom, or bathing. Adapted utensils, Velcro shoes, reachers, and bath chairs may be used. Your child's therapists can help you to choose appropriate equipment that is your child's size, meets his needs, and fits into your family's lifestyle.

Because a child's job is to play, assistive technology is also available for toys. Many toys may not need to be adapted for your child. Toys that combine sounds, sights, textures, and learning are ideal for any child. Some toys will need to be modified so that your child can play with them. A simple switch can be hooked up to a battery-operated toy and placed next to your child so that he can make a toy dog bark or a toy car drive. Switch-adapted toys can give a child with movement problems the opportunity to control something in his world. This can be a tremendous lift to a child's self-confidence.

Other types of toys can be modified for children with disabilities. Examples include tricycles with adapted foot straps or hand pedals, or a mechanical page turner for books that might also have large print. Many computer games and programs can be used by children with cerebral palsy. Key 29 provides other suggestions for helping your child play. You can also ask your child's case manager, teachers, or therapists about toy lending libraries that may be available in your community.

As your child grows up, access to recreation and leisure activities will become more important. Assistive technology may help him participate in recreation. Many people with disabilities, including some who walk most of the time, use lightweight wheelchairs to play sports like basketball or tennis. Board games, video games, stereos, TVs, and other leisure equipment can also be modified for your child.

Using adapted toys can lead to other important skills that allow your child to do more things on his own. Assistive technology can enhance mobility. Children learn through exploration. A baby crawls or toddles to discover his world. If your child with cerebral palsy cannot move his body very well, he may be able to explore using a scooter board, modified tricycle, or wheelchair. Using assistive technology for movement early in life does not necessarily mean that your child will never learn to walk. A wheelchair may substitute for walking until your child is strong enough and coordinated enough to walk on his own. A wheelchair may also become your child's only form of independent movement. If he cannot push a wheelchair, your child may be able to drive a power or motorized wheelchair with his hand by using a joystick or with his head or elbow by using an adapted switch. Hand controls or other adaptations are also available for automobiles if your child should find this helpful as a teenager or adult.

Assistive technology can also open up the world of communication for children with cerebral palsy. Although many people with cerebral palsy can speak clearly, some are not easy to understand. Others cannot speak at all. A speech language pathologist may work with your child to help him learn to communicate using assistive technology. *Augmentative or alternative communication* (AAC) may be as simple as pictures of familiar objects that your child can point to when he wants the object. The communication boards discussed in Key 42 are a good example. A tape recorder is another simple form of an AAC device. A child pushes an adapted switch to activate the tape recorder and "say" a prerecorded message. An AAC device can also be a box with a photograph or real object in each of four compartments. The child could scan through the four choices with a roaming light and hit an adapted switch when the light gets to the chosen item.

Your child may also learn to communicate using more complicated forms of technology depending on his abilities. Many people communicate with personal computers or laptop computers that have special programs and voices. Your child can use an adapted switch and scanner on the computer to select words or phrases to say. He might also directly press the keys one by one or even type whole messages. He can then hit a button and hear himself "talk" through the computer. This type of technology might be used by your child to complete homework, sing in a choir, or answer the telephone.

*Accessibility* is another area through which your child may be aided by assistive technology. Ramps, elevators, and wider doorways will make his life easier if he uses a wheelchair. You might find it helpful to arrange your home so that your child can do things more independently. Low pile carpet or vinyl flooring might make it easier to walk or push a wheelchair. Touch lamps may be more simple for your child to operate than light switches. Safety grab bars might be necessary in the bathroom. As your child grows up, simple adaptations and complicated modifications can be made to increase his ability to do more on his own. These might include lever door handles, large push buttons on the telephone or remote

## WHAT IS ASSISTIVE TECHNOLOGY?

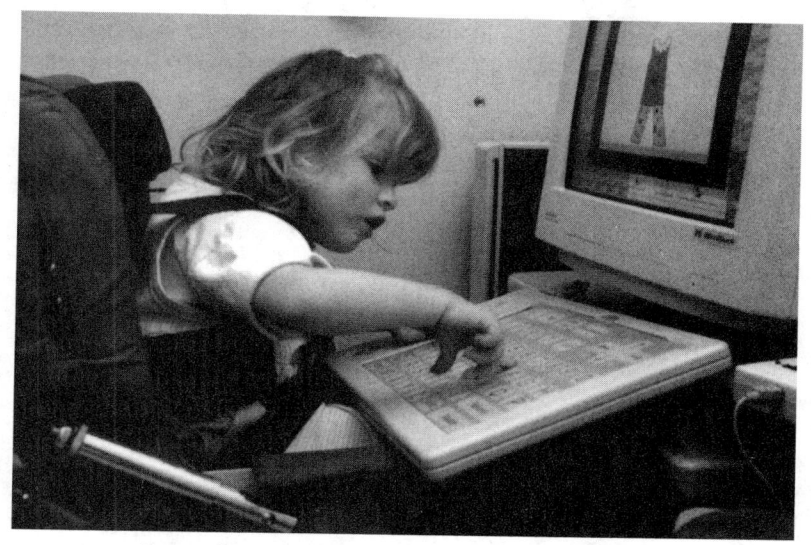

**Learning to use a keyboard and computer**

control, adapted kitchen or laundry facilities, mechanical lifts, and environmental controls for operating electronic devices like stereos from a power wheelchair.

Assistive technology can, in many cases, help a child, adolescent, or adult with cerebral palsy to do things others do without help. Assistive technology can help your child reach a higher level of independence and can greatly increase his self-confidence and quality of life. The resources section of this book lists manufacturers of different types of assistive technology. Before purchasing equipment, discuss your child's needs with his therapists. You may also need a doctor's prescription. Gather information from manufacturers, rehabilitation specialists, medical supply store personnel, and other parents. Bargain shop and let your child try out the equipment, especially wheelchairs and AAC devices. Some clinics, lending libraries, stores, and parent support groups share equipment. Take advantage of these options for your child.

# PART SEVEN

## YOUR CHILD'S FUTURE

This final section of the book contains many important issues to consider throughout your child's life. Planning for your child's future should start immediately. Part Seven gives suggestions for helping your child to build friendships, find interests, and set goals. You will also find compassionate advice for dealing with sex issues. This includes appropriate self-exploration, mature relationships, and safeguarding against abuse.

Part Seven stresses the importance of balancing finances and seeking funding assistance. It talks about guardianship, living arrangements, employment options, marriage, and moving from one stage in life to the next using transition planning. The final Key, "Letting Go," offers encouragement for allowing your child to spread his wings and fly.

# 44

# YOUR CHILD CAN MAKE FRIENDS

Making friends is important for all children. Inclusion programs in public schools that bring children with and without disabilities together provide new challenges and opportunities for friendships. Children with cerebral palsy, like all kids, need friends to help them build the emotional bridges from preschool to school-age to adolescence and into adulthood.

An important first step is to bring your child into the community. Often, a child's first contact with the larger world is school. Consider visiting your child's school a day or two before your child's enrollment. Bring pictures or a home video. Provide the children with a simple explanation of your child's disability. Bring along any special equipment that your child uses such as a wheelchair, braces, crutches, or a communication device so the children can see them, touch them, and ask questions. Before school starts, help your child practice introducing herself using her voice or communication device. Help your child develop a simple explanation for her disability and to act out appropriate ways to respond if she is teased.

You can do many things to make your home comfortable and inviting for children of all abilities to play together and build friendships. Adapt your home with ramps or grab bars that allow your child to move more easily and independently at home in order to keep up with other children in play activities. Keep a spare wheelchair or an extra pair of crutches to allow children to participate equally in obstacle courses, wheelchair sports, or crutch races. Provide books and toys that display children with disabilities in a positive light. Some commercial dolls now feature hearing aides or a wheelchair. Talk with your orthotist or therapist about tiny braces, crutches, or casts for a favorite doll. Encourage sleepovers, pizza parties, and listening to music with friends. Look for games and toys your child plays well. Do not feel that children have to be exactly the same age to play together. Some children with cerebral palsy play well with younger children who have similar developmental skills. Other children with cerebral palsy play better with an older child who perhaps is more calm, quiet, and patient.

Some families report their child's social opportunities were greatly increased by obtaining one unusual toy that attracted a large number of neighborhood children. Some families have built a special playhouse, added a sand or water table in the backyard, bought a Ping-Pong or pool table, purchased a video game, or added an outdoor pool to create a popular gathering place for new friends. Frequently taking your child to the neighborhood park can also spark new friendships.

Other children with cerebral palsy have built a network of good friends through joining a church or service group. Church youth groups and scouting offer structured activities and a nurturing environment in which to build friendships. Some areas have scouting troops for children with special needs. Adapted sports, such as wheelchair tennis or basketball, or Special Olympics can provide a lifetime of friendships, challenges, and opportunities for your child. Many parents have worked hard to network with other families of children with disabilities and formed informal play groups for their children. A parent support group can be a great place to start a children's play group.

Animals, especially gentle family pets, can be faithful friends to children with cerebral palsy. Even children with the most severe disabilities become calm, quiet, alert, and fascinated when holding a warm, furry animal in their arms. Animals are faithful friends who never tire of playing with a child and never criticize or tease. Learning to care for a pet lovingly can teach a child with cerebral palsy important life skills. Breeding, training, or showing a pet may provide tremendous social and vocational opportunities. Many children with cerebral palsy can become much more independent with carefully trained dogs, similar to those who assist people who are blind. A service dog can help a person with a disability in many ways and become a lifelong friend.

As your child looks for an opportunity to make friends, encourage activities or hobbies that minimize your child's disabilities and build on her strengths and interests. Symphonic band, choir, home economics, chess club, reading club, science fiction club, yearbook, photography, and other hobbies may be creative ways to meet and interact successfully with friends. Do not let your fear as a parent limit your child's social life. With a little planning and forethought, your child's life can be rich with friends and fun.

# 45

# DEVELOPING YOUR CHILD'S INTERESTS

Helping your child with cerebral palsy develop interests is crucial to helping him fully develop his personality. Interests frequently lead to hobbies, and hobbies can lead to satisfying work. Satisfying work is an important step toward independence.

The first step in helping your child to develop interests is giving him opportunities to make choices. Let your young child make some decisions about what he eats, drinks, wears, and plays. As he grows older, give him the responsibility of choosing his wardrobe and picking things to do in his leisure or free time. By learning to make choices, children not only gain some freedom but also learn what they like.

Next, find out what your child likes. Ask your child what he thinks is fun. What would he like to learn to do? Does he like to listen to music or stories? Is he a cartoon buff? Does he like to tell jokes? What types of programs interest him on television? Sports? Animals? Cooking shows? Car racing? Any of these interests can be expanded and adapted for your child with cerebral palsy.

If you are uncertain what your child really enjoys, expose him to a wide variety of interesting activities. Take him to a zoo, the museum, a car dealership, an airport, a live sporting event, a symphony, and so on. When possible, introduce him to the people who work and play in these settings. If your child seems excited or asks for a return visit, you have found an interest that can be developed. Your child may enjoy taking swimming or dancing lessons.

## DEVELOPING YOUR CHILD'S INTERESTS

Scouting programs for both boys and girls explore a wide variety of possible interests by having young people earn merit badges. Scouting is an organized way to meet other young people and explore many different interests from camping to music. Your child can also find things he likes through his siblings, friends, and school. Remember that the interests you are developing are your child's rather than your own. Do not dampen his enthusiasm for rap or country music just because you do not enjoy it.

Once you have identified an interest, help your child learn about it. Read books or magazines to your child about his interest. In many cases, your child can learn more by joining a club with people who share similar interests. Reading books, writing poetry, photography, cooking, art, music, or science fiction do not really require mobility skills and can be good choices for adults and children with cerebral palsy. The Internet can also provide a way for children with cerebral palsy to hook up with other people who share their interests. Children with cerebral palsy can type or use specially adapted equipment to communicate through a computer. This levels the playing field for a child whose speech is difficult to understand or who has difficulty with movement.

Look for a mentor for your child. Meeting a teenager or adult who has experience or special skills in your child's area of interest can be a life changing opportunity for your child. Teenagers, college students, or retired people can often find the time to teach a special skill to your child that can provide him with a lifetime of enjoyment.

If possible, you can travel to help explore your child's interest area. Traveling to a special convention, exhibit, performance, or concert dealing with your child's favorite interest can really be a wonderful growth experience. Having experience traveling to an unfamiliar place, meeting new people, and being away from home and family can really bolster your child's confidence. This shows him that he can be more independent.

Adapt an interest or hobby so that your child with cerebral palsy can be successful with it. Perhaps your child's interest is tennis. In the beginning, you may be very sad that he cannot just jump up and play tennis professionally. However, your child can watch and enjoy tennis on television, travel to various tennis tournaments, collect memorabilia about tennis, read books about tennis, work one-on-one with a tennis coach learning how to hit the ball, keep score for or make videos of the school tennis team, use an adapted racquet to play, or start a wheelchair tennis team. Think about all the things your child can do rather than the things he cannot do.

If your child's interests change, drop an activity and move on. All children go through stages where they are passionately interested in an activity and then leave it to pursue something else. If your child's hobby requires a great deal of time and expense, pursue the hobby for a set length of time and then reevaluate whether he wants to continue it. Musical, sports, and other equipment can often be borrowed or rented. This gives a child more room to explore with less expense if he changes his mind. With a little creativity, you can help your child with cerebral palsy develop interests that will give him a lifetime of enjoyment and, perhaps, more independence for work and play.

# 46

# DEVELOPING REALISTIC GOALS

One of the most challenging tasks for parents raising a child with cerebral palsy is to help their child and the team of professionals set realistic goals. This is often a difficult task for parents. Sometimes, parents just do not know what realistically to expect their child to accomplish. Some parents expect their child to function completely normally despite severe brain damage. Other parents underestimate what their child can do.

One of the most important things you can do is to discover and nurture your child's interests. Your child's own goals are very important. Even when your child is very young, it may be very obvious that she desperately wants to feed herself without your help or wants to learn to crawl to keep up with other children. A child is much more likely to accomplish a goal that is important to her. Some children with cerebral palsy will focus very strongly on learning to ride a tricycle or bicycle. Some teenagers will want to try out for the school band or drama club. Some are intensely focused on earning a high school diploma. Just remember your child's goals and dreams are the most important issue. Your goals and dreams for your child take second place to hers.

Always build on your child's strengths and interests. If you set goals based on your child's strengths and potential, she can more successfully learn skills that lead to future employment, living on her own, or having an enjoyable hobby.

Goals should include your child's desires but also be realistic. If your child has a goal that seems unrealistic, be creative and come up with ways to achieve it, at least to some extent. For example, suppose your sixteen-year-old daughter who must use a wheelchair wants to be a pilot. Set small goals that can be easily achieved and are steps toward a bigger goal. Goals might include learning about flying by reading books and meeting pilots, visiting airports, and finding jobs in the flight industry that are accessible to her. Perhaps your child could take flying lessons if she has good use of her hands and good mental abilities. Through ingenuity, you can help your child realistically meet her goals.

When you set a small goal you should always be certain that it moves toward the bigger, long-term goal. For example, assume that your long-term goal is that your child will be able to sit up on the floor by herself. An appropriate short-term goal might be that in two months, she will sit with her hands propped on the floor for support while listening to a short song like *London Bridge*. As your child improves, her next short-term goal might be to do the same skill throughout longer songs. A later stage might be to sit with her hands off the floor while playing pat-a-cake. This demands greater balance.

An action plan is a way to map out strategies for achieving a goal. It may be part of the training plans discussed in Key 38 or something your family develops individually. In an action plan, the goal is written in specific, measurable terms and specifies a time frame to meet the goals. Designate activities appropriate for achieving the goal and address the following questions: When and where will the child work on the goal? Who will gather the results of your child's progress? How will results be recorded? How long will your child work on this goal? How will the team measure whether or not the child has succeeded or failed? How will changes be made in the strategies? Is the goal functional and meaningful? Does it improve your child's independence? Does it make your child feel better about herself? Is the goal a logical step toward an important larger goal? Is this goal important to you and your child at this time? Do you have the resources needed such as therapy, time, or special equipment to accomplish this particular goal? Reevaluating and updating goals regularly gives your child the best opportunity to make progress.

**DEVELOPING REALISTIC GOALS**

Have your child's physician, therapist, teacher, or even another experienced parent of a child with cerebral palsy review and critique your child's goals. Often, their opinions can help you decide what is most important for your child. Another person's viewpoint can help you set priorities and keep you from losing precious time working on a goal that is not realistic, not functional, or just plain not important in your child's life.

Remember that your ultimate goal is for your child to do as many things as independently as possible. For a child to be able to communicate her wants and needs is often more important than being able to move by herself. If a computer, crutches, a wheelchair, or an electronic communication device make your child more independent and functional, the equipment should be used to its fullest extent in all settings. Looking ordinary is just not as important as being more functional and independent.

# 47

# MAKING A POSITIVE CONTRIBUTION TO SOCIETY

Your life and your child's life can either be devastated or be enhanced by dealing with the challenges of cerebral palsy. Whether you are devastated or enhanced is largely a choice. One of the most effective ways to regain purpose and control over your lives is to decide to do everything you can to make something positive come out of a difficult circumstance.

Everyone needs to feel useful, important, and valuable, like his life has made a difference. In order to have self-worth and self-esteem, people with cerebral palsy need to have an opportunity to make a positive contribution to society.

Christopher Reeve suffered a devastating spinal cord injury and is paralyzed. He cannot sit alone or use his hands, and has difficulty breathing for long periods without a respirator. Despite this, with his determined attitude, public appearances, and advocacy, Christopher Reeve has made a huge contribution to neurological research and has had a tremendous impact on the perceived value of people with disabilities in this society. Although wealthy and famous before his disability, he may have a much more important and profound positive impact on society after his injury. Gerry Jewel, an adult television and comedic actress with cerebral palsy, uses stand-up comedy as a vehicle to reach people and teach them about cerebral palsy through humor. Using her acting and comedy

## MAKING A POSITIVE CONTRIBUTION TO SOCIETY

talent, she has turned cerebral palsy into a professional asset. Gerry Jewel has made a conscious choice to make a positive out of a negative.

The first steps to helping your child make a positive contribution is to find, value, and use his strengths. Let your child know that every time he smiles, waves, or hugs someone, he is making a positive contribution to someone else's day. Your child should understand that his upbeat, optimistic, positive attitude can inspire and motivate other people. Give your child praise when he shows a positive attitude or tries to make someone happy.

Use your child's strengths, gifts, and talents to help him make a positive contribution to the community. Find a way for your child to serve others. Your child will grow greatly by having a chance to help other people who also have troubles. A wise saying is, "I cried because I had no shoes, until I met a man who had no feet."

With a little help from family or friends, all children with cerebral palsy can find a worthwhile way to serve others. Your child can visit elderly people in a nursing home, bringing cookies or flowers. He can help you gather toys or food for a homeless shelter. Maybe your child can read a story to other children at a library, hospital, or orphanage. Many children with cerebral palsy canvas their neighborhoods regularly in their wheelchairs with coffee cans in their laps to raise money for children with muscular dystrophy or to buy toys for disadvantaged children at Christmas. Many a hard heart has been deeply moved by their unselfish efforts. All these positive contributions by children with cerebral palsy should be encouraged.

Many children with cerebral palsy in the course of serving others have made friends and discovered talents they did not know they had. For some, those talents have developed into jobs, careers, lifelong friendships, and feelings of self-worth and confidence.

Your child can make other positive contributions besides public service. The challenges he faces may prompt his family members to become advocates for people who have disabilities. His friends, siblings, or classmates might choose their careers based on the impact he has had on their lives. His presence may improve the accessibility of his school for other students. His neighbors might think differently about disabilities. He might teach student therapists, doctors, or teachers a thing or two about cerebral palsy. Maybe he will be the first person with a disability to work for a particular company. Then again, his contributions to society might be as simple as holding any type of job, attending church, or voting for public officials. No matter what, your child with cerebral palsy makes a positive impact on the world just by being himself.

# 48

# TRANSITION: PLANNING FOR THE NEXT STEP

Life is a cycle of progressive steps. People naturally step from home to school, to work, to marriage and families, and, later, to retirement. Somehow, they make the transition from kindergarten to first grade and from living with their parents to living on their own. It probably took a certain amount of time and effort to make these steps easier because change is often difficult to handle.

People with disabilities usually need extra planning in order to step from one stage in life to another. *Transition planning* should occur between each major change in your child's life. This includes between early intervention and entering school, from elementary school to junior high and then high school, between school and work or higher education, and from the family home to your child's own home.

Transition planning plays such an important part in education that it is mandated in special education laws. Planning for the move from early intervention programs to school is required in individualized family services plans (IFSPs). This planning must occur when your child is two years old, if not before, because at the age of three, services are provided by the public school system. Make sure new team members are familiar with your child before the transition occurs. Consider ordering a wheelchair or mobility device, if necessary, so that your child can be transported by bus.

Contemplate ordering adaptive equipment, such as switch toys, and therapy equipment to use at home. You can prepare your child for this transition by visiting the school or day care setting, helping her feel comfortable around groups of children, and talking about what will happen in the new setting.

The *Individuals with Disabilities Education Act* (IDEA) of 1990 requires that transition plans be a part of individualized education programs (IEPs). As a member of your child's IEP team, you should make sure that planning occurs to help your child transition between different schools, teachers, and methods of transportation. The most important time for transition planning during the school years is several years before graduation. Make sure planning is started when your child is about fourteen years old in order to prepare for life after graduation.

Moving between school and adult services can be a very difficult time for people with disabilities and their families. Unfortunately, less services are available for people over the age of twenty-one. The services available for adults often have long waiting lists. Parents of younger and older adults with cerebral palsy may feel like they are crawling through an endless maze when it comes to adult services. This includes areas such as funding, healthcare, adaptive equipment, work, and living arrangements. The difficulty in acquiring adult services makes it all the more important for you to plan ahead so that the transition to adulthood is smooth and services are in place.

Some strategies help parents in the transition process: Have goals for your child's life in the community. Recognize the importance of your contributions as parents. Honor your child's choices. Make and use a network of social supports. Voice your concerns about future issues such as classroom placement, employment, and living arrangements.

Your participation in the transition process is key to ensuring that services are consistent and continuous for your child. Planning for upcoming life changes can make things go more smoothly. Remember that everyone finds change stressful. Careful transition planning can reduce the stress and make it less difficult for your child to take the steps needed to progress through life toward greater independence.

# 49

# GOING TO WORK

Schools are responsible for helping students with disabilities move from school into the adult worlds of higher education or employment. Teenagers with disabilities have been guaranteed vocational education opportunities through a 1990 law called the *Carl D. Perkins Vocational and Applied Technology Education Act*. Between the ages of fourteen and sixteen, your child should begin vocational education. Opportunities to try different job tasks or hold temporary community jobs through school will help your child to prepare for the world of work.

Right now, it might seem impossible that your child with cerebral palsy will ever hold a job. Truthfully, less than 20 percent of adults with cerebral palsy are competitively employed. However, the doors to employment for people with disabilities are being opened and expanded every day thanks to legislation such as the *Americans with Disabilities Act* and the creativity of teachers, job trainers, and parents. Imagination and resourcefulness are important ingredients in making job opportunities available for people with cerebral palsy.

Consider your daughter's or son's interests and abilities when developing an employment plan. If your child prefers standing to sitting and needs a lot of structure, doing graphic design on a computer might not fit his personality. Assembly work in a local business, however, may be right up your child's alley. Your child's competence in the following areas should also be considered for determining work placement and vocational training: attention span, safety habits, personal hygiene, transportation skills, time concepts, motor skills, ability to follow directions, money concepts, dressing skills, job interview skills, and social skills.

## Competitive Employment

Competitive employment means that the employee is in a competitive job market. He has the same responsibilities and earns the same salary as other workers with his job title. Some people with cerebral palsy complete college or vocational training programs and enter the workforce. An adult with cerebral palsy might work as an engineer, therapist, teacher, business manager, cook, janitor, or secretary, just to name a few possible career choices.

Certain factors increase the likelihood of a person with cerebral palsy holding a job. These include mild physical involvement, good family support, vocational training, and good employment contacts. Other factors contributing to independent employment include regular schooling, traveling independently beyond the home, good hand skills, living in a smaller community, and having spasticity rather than involuntary movements.

## Supported Employment

Supported employment involves assisting a person with a disability to locate, acquire, and learn a job. Agencies such as the Department of Vocational Rehabilitation provide supported employment. Vocational Rehabilitation is a cooperative federal-state program that performs an evaluation to determine a person's eligibility for the program. If eligible, goals and job options are determined with the help of vocational counselors. Other community agencies may provide supported employment also.

Through supported employment, job coaches are often provided to workers. A job coach helps a person with a disability to learn a community job. First, the job coach learns the job. On a one-to-one basis, he then teaches the employee the skills needed to perform the job. The job coach assists the worker as needed and gradually withdraws until the worker is independent. The job coach monitors the worker's progress and trains new skills as needed. In addition to this individualized form of supported employment, employees with disabilities may work together in a small group within a community job setting. The employees are trained and supervised as a group but also work with people who do not have disabilities.

Supported employment allows people with disabilities to work alongside workers without disabilities. These community jobs can be located with any employer willing to support a person with special needs. Examples include fast-food restaurants, retail stores, shopping malls, recycling centers, housekeeping services, schools, and hospitals. After conquering supported employment, the worker might be ready for competitive employment.

**Sheltered Workshops**

Sheltered workshops for people with cerebral palsy and other conditions are available in many communities. In a sheltered workshop, employees with disabilities usually perform repetitive tasks in supervised work stations. The tasks may be very simple such as sorting recyclable items, assembling parts for a contract, or making crafts to sell. The employee is paid a minimal wage often based on how long it takes to complete the task. Workers may also be paid for each completed product.

Sheltered workshops may be run by a community organization such as the Arc (formerly, the Association for Retarded Citizens), state institutions, or private businesses. A sheltered workshop may be a stepping stone toward supported or competitive employment much like a summer job is for a high school student. The workshop can also be a more permanent job placement for individuals with challenging behaviors, lower mental abilities, or more severe physical impairments. Remember that sheltered workshops allow workers to earn some money, gain work skills, and develop self-esteem.

**Work Activity Centers and Adult Day Care Programs**

Some people with cerebral palsy may not develop basic skills for holding a job. Work activity centers or adult day care programs can provide these individuals with adult activities that encourage social, self-help, and leisure skills. Prevocational and vocational training is provided, but wages are not earned. These centers provide an important function in society because they allow adults with severe disabilities an opportunity to socialize and do something meaningful. Quite possibly, some of these people could develop skills that would allow them to transition into the workforce.

## Resources

Resources for employment vary from state to state. Examples include a Department of Vocational Rehabilitation, the Arc, Goodwill Industries, a state employment office, a job training partnership act (JTPA), and local colleges or universities. Some employment resources are listed in the back of this book.

# 50

# HANDLING SEX EDUCATION

It is difficult for any parent to acknowledge a child's journey through sexual development. This journey differs for every family, largely depending on your child's mental and physical abilities and personality. Every family needs to consider some common issues.

All humans are sexual beings. Even children with severe mental and physical disabilities need to be touched, held, and cuddled. Children with cerebral palsy, like all children, will, to the best of their ability, explore all parts of their bodies. They need to be given names for their body parts and an explanation of their functions. Most children with cerebral palsy, except some who have difficulty tolerating physical touch, will experience normal feelings of sexual arousal if touched in sensitive areas. A child with cerebral palsy who occasionally touches his penis or her vagina is normal. This is only a problem for the family if the child touches himself or herself over and over or if the child touches his or her private parts in public. If the child can understand, it is important to explain that it is acceptable to touch her body but only in a private room. If your child masturbates in public, offer a toy or activity, remind the child that touching her body is only for private time, or take the child to a private area. It is fine to tell your child "no" and that her behavior is *not appropriate* in public. It is not helpful to yell, threaten, or physically punish a child for the normal exploration of the body.

Sometimes in cases of severe brain damage, children masturbate a great deal of the time and show little interest in toys or activities intended to distract them. Frequently, it is helpful to clap the child's hands together rhythmically, rock the child in your arms, sing to the child, or help the child hold a toy or stuffed animal in her hands to help her focus on other sensations, sights, or sounds.

In children who have cerebral palsy, the timing of puberty can vary widely. Some children with cerebral palsy, for reasons not understood, have a condition called precocious puberty. In precocious puberty, boys grow tall, develop facial and body hair, have their voices deepen, and sometimes develop acne before they reach their teenage years. In girls with precocious puberty, they grow tall, may develop acne, may begin their menstrual period, develop body hair, and develop breast buds before their teenage years. Signs of early or late puberty should always be evaluated by a doctor. Other children with cerebral palsy may begin adolescent body changes later than their peers. Children with delayed physical growth in height and weight may be more likely to enter puberty late. Medication and the location of brain damage may also play a role.

An important part of helping your child with cerebral palsy manage sexual development well is doing everything possible to make your child independent at keeping her body clean. A young person with cerebral palsy will feel much more confident and good about herself if she is as independent as possible in bathing, dressing, and using the toilet. Special adapted equipment, medications, and sometimes surgeries to release tight hip muscles or to help improve bowel and bladder control can make a tremendous difference. Ask your child's doctor or therapist about a bladder or bowel management program for your child. Many children with mild or moderate cerebral palsy, even with moderate mental retardation, can be toilet trained successfully. Do not just assume that your child will wear diapers all her life. A careful professional plan is absolutely necessary.

Young women with cerebral palsy and their families will face the task of managing a menstrual period. Learning to manage pads and tampons is a skill that some young women have to practice patiently. This is especially true if they have difficulty balancing while sitting or using their hands well.

Another important responsibility for parents of children with cerebral palsy is to help safeguard your child against sexual abuse. If your child with cerebral palsy cannot communicate verbally, your child will require more protection against possible sexual abuse from caregivers, classmates, strangers, and family acquaintances. The best protection for a child who cannot talk is the careful supervision of a loving parent or a trusted longtime caregiver. Parents cannot realistically supervise a person with cerebral palsy twenty-four hours per day forever, so other protection must be developed.

Choose your baby-sitters, group homes, hospitals, residential settings, rehabilitation programs, home health care agencies, and camps carefully. Never allow anyone to care for your child before you have checked references. Do not rely on written references. Insist on a current phone number where you can speak directly to the patient or family the employee took care of. Talking to the supervisor of the employee is not enough. If the person you are hiring works for an agency or facility, ask if and when a criminal background check was run on the employee. Ask if any complaints have been filed against the employee. If the company or agency does not run criminal checks on its employees, look for another company. Your local health department can often provide information about health care agencies in your area. Ask to see reports from their inspections or accreditation visits. Many of these records are available through the *Freedom of Information Act*. Another source of information about possible abuse is the State Attorney General's office.

If your child can speak, teach your child that her body is private. Empower your child to say "no" and yell for help if anyone touches her body in a way that makes her feel uncomfortable. Listen carefully to your child and reassure her that you will always believe her. Preprogram your phone to dial 911 and your work number or a trusted neighbor's number. Encourage your child to use the phone to call for help anytime she feels endangered. Trust your instincts. If you are not comfortable with the caregiver, do not leave your child. Watch your caregiver and your child interact together. Keep your first few stays together short so you can check in on your child frequently. Give your child a code word such as "purple shoes" she can use as a private signal to let you know over the phone that something is wrong. This lets you know that you need to come home immediately or call 911. A child with cerebral palsy talking to mom over the phone can say, "Mom, have you seen my purple shoes?" and not arouse suspicion. Code words work better than saying, "My baby-sitter just hit me or fondled me or scared me, and I need help." A careful plan such as this will help protect your child against physical or sexual abuse.

Every parent of a teenager faces complex issues as the child matures into adolescence and young adulthood. For most teenagers, some of the growing up lessons are taught by parents, and some lessons are taught by schoolmates and friends. For some children with cerebral palsy, parents will do more of the teaching because a child with cerebral palsy may not have any friends with similar special needs. For teenagers with cerebral palsy, parents need to be prepared to teach their children about privacy, modesty, and sexually appropriate behavior.

Preteens and teenagers need to know how their bodies work. Your child needs to understand that feelings of sexual attraction are healthy and normal. Teach her the facts about sex and reproduction. Many teenagers with cerebral palsy date. Some date people with disabilities, and others date people without disabilities. Your child needs to know that expressions of sexual behavior are only appropriate between consenting adults. Teach her that with sexual activity comes adult responsibility. Sexually transmitted disease, AIDS, safe sex, birth control, and pregnancy all need to be thoroughly discussed at your child's level of understanding. The depth and complexity of these discussions increases as your child grows older.

The information detailed in this Key should help you to be better prepared and more comfortable in teaching your child to handle this challenging time of change.

# 51

# SEXUALITY, MARRIAGE, AND PARENTHOOD

Many young adults with cerebral palsy can look forward to satisfying adult friendships, sexual relationships, marriage, and parenthood. Careful adult problem solving and planning should be part of each maturation step.

People with cerebral palsy usually have normal sensation throughout their bodies. This means that the feelings associated with sexual enjoyment including arousal, lubrication, orgasm, and ejaculation are the same as in people without cerebral palsy. A person with cerebral palsy experiencing a sexual difficulty should be treated and evaluated very thoroughly, because a difficulty often signals a problem not connected to cerebral palsy.

Tight arm and leg muscles, poor balance, difficulty in hand function, and poor coordination can create challenges for people with cerebral palsy in expressing themselves sexually. Sometimes, medication or surgery that addresses tight muscles, or special pillows and positioning equipment can help. Typically, most people with cerebral palsy have more movement and coordination difficulty if they are nervous, stressed, cold, or in a hurry and try to move too quickly. A warm, relaxing atmosphere with good, secure positioning and a patient, gentle partner will provide the best environment for a satisfying sexual relationship.

Birth control and protection against sexually transmitted disease should not be overlooked. Young adults with cerebral palsy should be fully involved in and fully informed about making these types of decisions. Parents and young adults with cerebral palsy should be aware that only latex condoms offer protection against sexually transmitted disease; other birth control methods do not. Some people with cerebral palsy may have a latex allergy. If so, they should not use any item containing latex including latex condoms and diaphragms. Your child's physician, gynecologist, or urologist can be very helpful in dealing with the issues of birth control and sexually transmitted disease.

It is important that teenagers and adults with cerebral palsy receive the same routine reproductive healthcare as anyone else. Routine breast examination, mammography, pap smears, treatment of vaginal or urinary tract infections, colorectal exams, testicular and prostate exams, and evaluation of symptoms of genitourinary burning, itching, redness, and discharge are just as important as for a nondisabled person. Finding a urologist or gynecologist who is gentle, sensitive, and works frequently with people who have disabilities is important. Large adult rehabilitation centers or university hospitals can often be useful in finding helpful medical specialists.

Many adults with cerebral palsy will consider marriage at some point in their lives. Young adults and their families thinking about the future need to remember that decisions about marrying and becoming parents are separate. When contemplating marriage, a person should thoughtfully consider several questions. Am I in love with this individual? Are we ready to make a lifetime commitment to one another? How well do we handle problems together? Are we independent enough to live on our own? Do we need attendant care? Do we have a safe, secure, accessible place to live? Do we have the money, jobs, transportation, and medical care that we will need? Have I had enough dating experience to know that this person is a good life partner? Do I or my future spouse have serious medical, lifestyle, or emotional problems that would make marriage difficult? Whether or not one or both of the partners has cerebral palsy or any other disability is not nearly as important as the answers to these very important questions.

Women with cerebral palsy are typically physically capable of becoming pregnant and carrying a baby to term unless they have some other medical complication. Special care may need to be taken to prevent falls during pregnancy that might harm the unborn child. Men with cerebral palsy are typically capable of having sexual relations and fathering children unless they have another unrelated medical problem.

The decision whether or not to become a parent is one of the most serious decisions any adult can make. The future of a vulnerable child is at stake. Any child will be completely dependent on its parents for care. Men and women with cerebral palsy have the same desires to be parents as anyone else. Those desires should be honored and respected.

The right for a person with cerebral palsy to have children is protected by law like any other citizen. No one can give a person temporary or permanent birth control or sterilization without the person's informed consent. If someone with cerebral palsy cannot give informed consent for temporary or permanent birth control or sterilization, the consent cannot be given by parents or guardians without due legal process.

Parents of all children have the important responsibility of helping their teenagers and young adults understand that being a parent is a huge, long-term responsibility. Many people with cerebral palsy are excellent, competent parents. They should ask themselves: Am I in a stable, loving relationship? Are both partners ready to share the responsibility of raising a child? Am I physically capable of holding, feeding, carrying, diapering, and supervising a young child? Can a wheelchair or other special equipment help me do this? Do I have accessible housing for myself and my family? Do I have adequate money, transportation, and health care for myself and my family? Do I have the attendant care that I will need? Will I need extended family support to raise a child? Do I have a network of family and friends that I can depend on to help with child care? Do my spouse, family, and friends generally support the idea of my becoming a parent? Do I have any special medical problems or take any medication that should be taken into consideration? Do I have the symptoms of cerebral palsy because of a genetic or chromosomal abnormality? Do we need genetic counseling? By carefully considering these questions, your adult child can make the best decisions about raising a family.

The journey through sexual development is long and sometimes complex. With planning, education, sensitivity, and open communication, it can be a fulfilling aspect of life for your loved one with cerebral palsy.

# 52

# PLACES TO LIVE

Through support from family, friends, early intervention, school services, and the medical community, you may have been able to care for your child at home. It may have been a struggle, but you, your child, and your family have benefitted from creating a home together.

Perhaps you chose to have your child grow up somewhere other than your home. It is often difficult for families to stay together as a unit when a family member has a disability. For whatever reason, your child may live in a state facility or institution, a home for children with disabilities, a foster care setting, or a relative's home. If you have remained your child's guardian or advocate, you should be actively involved in decisions regarding where your child lives and the care he receives.

At some point, children grow up and leave home. Having a child with cerebral palsy will complicate the issue. Transition from the family home to another home will take more time. Just like finding employment for your child, seeking options for living arrangements requires time and commitment.

Living arrangements vary from community to community. Options range from completely independent living to institutionalization. In the past, parents of children with cerebral palsy were encouraged to send their children away to institutions or state schools. This was considered the best way to care for people who were retarded or disabled. Today, parents are encouraged to keep their children at home or find a living arrangement other than the more restrictive environment of an institution. In recent years, there has been a push for people with cerebral palsy to live in their local community. This is called community integration. Rather than isolating people, the focus is on providing opportunities to live, work, and socialize with people who do not have disabilities.

**Independent Living**

Independent living, as the name implies, means a person does not need supervision in order to take care of himself or his affairs. He manages his money, his home, and his job without help. It is possible that your child with cerebral palsy will live on his own as an adult. It may take considerable planning, training, and assistive technology for your child to be independent, but it is a possibility. If your child is able to live independently, he will continue to need parental support just like anybody else. Do not be afraid to let him leave the nest; he will always need your love and caring guidance.

**Semi-Independent Living**

Semi-independent living, in one form, is much like a college dormitory or retirement home. Residents in a program live alone or with roommates in apartment complexes. The apartments are usually designed for people with disabilities. The programs offer a certain amount of help with money management, employment, community involvement, and other similar services. Mostly though, the residents fend for themselves, including cooking and cleaning.

Another type of semi-independent living is provided through adult companion programs. An adult with cerebral palsy lives with an adult roommate who does not have a disability. The roommate volunteers to participate in the program, provides support as needed, and allows the person with cerebral palsy to be as independent as possible.

**Special Foster Care**

Special foster care is an option for children and adults with disabilities. Foster care providers are trained to take care of someone who has a disability. They receive payment for room and board and for caring for the child or adult with cerebral palsy. Foster care provides a family and home setting as well as training for the child.

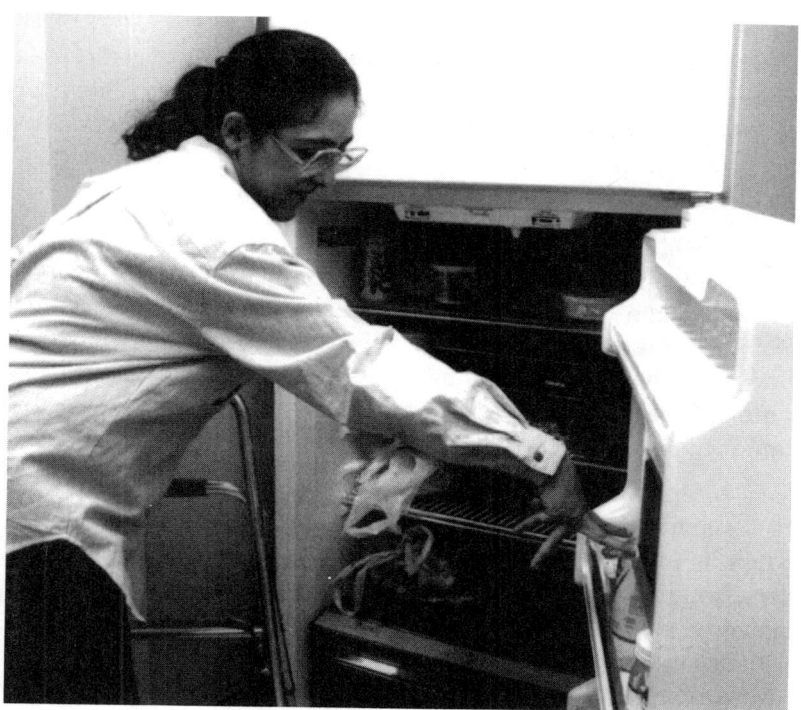

Getting a snack

## Shared Living

In shared living arrangements, two to three people with varying degrees of disabilities share a home and support staff. The staff might include two or more personal care attendants or habilitation aides and a home manager. Usually, the attendants assist the residents with daily needs and with learning skills to promote independence. The home manager takes care of cooking and cleaning. Most of the time, the staff is provided and supervised by a private company or state agency. The residents in shared living arrangements participate in school or work and in community activities. Sometimes, several parents of adult children with cerebral palsy jointly purchase a home for their children to share.

## Group Homes

Usually five to six people with disabilities live together in a group home. They may share a room and share responsibilities for daily routines like cooking dinner or cleaning. Similar to shared living arrangements, staff provide care and training in group homes. Again, the staff is supervised by a company or agency.

## Residential Settings

Residential settings are large centers that care for many children or adults with all types of disabilities. A nursing home is an example of a residential setting. Although some people with cerebral palsy live in nursing homes, this is usually far from an ideal setting. Care is not always appropriate for their age or abilities, and training in independent skills is often not provided.

Intermediate care facilities and state institutions are large residential settings that take care of many people with disabilities. Often, between 50 and 500 residents may live there. Intermediate care facilities are run by private companies and sometimes have a sheltered workshop for residents. Institutions or state schools are usually larger and are run by state agencies. Both types of settings provide care and training for the residents. State institutions, however, are being reduced in size all over the country as residents are moved into smaller, more homelike environments. This is called *deinstitutionalization*.

All of the living arrangement options listed in this Key, as well as your family home, can provide safe, appropriate care for your son or daughter with cerebral palsy. Supervision is provided in all of the options to ensure that the residents are cared for correctly. Some of the options are more isolating than others. For example, institutions usually exist on the outside of towns, whereas shared living arrangements are within more typical neighborhoods.

When trying to decide where your child will live now or as an adult, be sure that you consider his desires and training needs. Today, none of the options have to be permanent. Therefore, your child can move from one setting to another, especially if he becomes more independent.

# 53

# MEETING YOUR FINANCIAL NEEDS

Few things cause as many worries as financial burdens. The medical, therapeutic, and equipment needs of a child with cerebral palsy will stretch your finances, possibly to their limits. Many of these expenses may be tax deductible and/or covered by your medical insurance. Unfortunately, you will still have to come up with part, if not all, of the money up front. Additionally, a large number of children do not have insurance and are in families with low income.

If your child was hospitalized for an extended period of time at birth because of her medical problems, someone from the hospital should have spoken with you about finances. Your medical expenses, especially if your child was in a neonatal intensive care unit (NICU), could be astronomical. It is hoped that a case manager was assigned to your child, and you discussed your financial situation, insurance coverage, and other funding options. Do you already have a game plan?

If not, it is time to get a case manager. If your child is under three years old, place her in an early intervention (EI) program, and use the EI case manager. A case manager should be on your child's team at school, whether she is in regular or special education classes. If your child is not in early intervention or school, a case manager should be available through other appropriate programs such as your state Departments of Health, Vocational Rehabilitation, or Education. Social workers or rehabilitation program personnel can also serve as case managers.

The importance of a case manager is stressed because this person, more than anyone else, is responsible for finding and coordinating resources and services for your child. Your child's therapists, nurses, and other professionals as well as other parents of children with disabilities can be valuable resources, too. These people often collect information on financial and other resources for families.

You should also research funding sources for your child. If a professional tells you that Medicaid will not cover a piece of equipment, like a special car seat, ask for suggestions of other car seat providers, like Easter Seals, perhaps. If your insurance company denies coverage on a service or a piece of equipment, do not take "no" for an answer. Put up a fight. Ask your child's physician and therapists for letters of medical necessity explaining the benefit of the requested equipment or service. A heartfelt letter from a parent can also influence an insurance company or agency's decision.

If your attempts at financial assistance fail, ask for a payment plan from the service or equipment provider. You might be able to pay for some equipment on layaway. You can also check with the Rehabilitation Engineering and Assistive Technology Society of North America (RESNA) for equipment recycling programs in your area. Lastly, you could put a little money at a time into a savings account to purchase necessary or desired items for your child.

It would be impossible to discuss every type of financial assistance program available to people with cerebral palsy in this Key. Many are listed in the resource section of this book. Often, you will find that contacting one resource uncovers several other options. Keep a list in your child's care notebook because you never know when you will need options for yourself or other families. Although every family's situation is different, some financial assistance information can be generalized across the United States.

**Insurance**
Keep your child's special needs in mind when deciding on the type and provider of medical and dental insurance. Read your policy and find out what is and is not covered. Make sure services are

authorized before they are started. This can keep you from paying the whole bill. File a claims appeal with the company if it denies coverage. Use letters of medical necessity.

## Government Agencies

### Department of Education

Education and related services are free by law. Equipment listed in a child's IEP (individualized education program) and shown to meet a need related to a child's education may be paid for by the local school district.

### Departments of Health, Human Services, or Developmental Disabilities

The specific name of the agency varies from state to state. A variety of services may be available depending on your income. These include community-based alternatives to nursing home placement, respite, home care, habilitation, durable medical and therapeutic equipment, medical supplies, certain living expenses, therapy, and support services.

### Department of Vocational Rehabilitation

"Voc. Rehab." provides job training, placement, and support as well as funding for equipment necessary for a person with a disability to hold a job.

## Medicaid and Medicare

These federal health insurance programs may be available to people with a disability or a chronic disease, depending on the family's income. They cover medically related expenses like surgery, medication, hospitalization, supplies, equipment, and therapy. People under the age of twenty-one are eligible for Medicaid. Those over twenty years old who receive Social Security disability benefits can qualify for Medicare. U.S. citizenship may be necessary for services. Some states have other programs for which non-U.S. citizens can apply.

## Social Security Administration

Supplemental Security Income (SSI) benefits for children with disabilities are available through Social Security. SSI adds to the income of families with children under eighteen years old. If your income is too high to qualify your child for SSI benefits, your child may qualify after her eighteenth birthday, because her income is then considered separate from the family's. SSI benefits may also be available to children of adults receiving social security benefits. Check with your local social security office for details. The social security office may refer your child to a Children with Special Health Care Needs (CSHCN) program provided through your state. You can contact local hospitals, social service offices, or health departments for information.

**Grants**

A grant is basically a request for funding that becomes a payment source once the grant is approved. Sometimes, the government, corporations, and individuals provide money as grants to fund certain programs. Often, an organization or a university writes and handles grants for people with disabilities.

**Associations and Charities**

The United Cerebral Palsy Association (UCPA), the Arc, the Easter Seals Society, the March of Dimes, Shriner's Orthopedic Hospitals, and other similar organizations may also provide financial assistance to people with cerebral palsy. Asking other parents of children with cerebral palsy about funding sources and financial assistance programs may be your best bet. They may have found supportive people in charity organizations, parent groups, or government programs. Other parents have been where you now are and can help you find your way through the funding maze.

# 54

# FINANCIAL PLANNING AND GUARDIANSHIP

In addition to the everyday concerns of parenthood, parents have to plan for the future. This includes making sure that enough money is available to pay for future needs and that the children will be taken care of when the parents are no longer living. Planning is extremely important for families of children with cerebral palsy.

Financial planning comes in many forms. Ask advice from a professional financial planner, preferably one with experience in disability issues. This Key contains some basic suggestions for financial planning.

Look into financial assistance programs that are available in your community, in your state, and at the national level. If your child qualifies, be sure to keep the paperwork up-to-date so his coverage does not lapse. If he does not qualify now, check again in the future when he is an adult or if your financial situation changes. Other programs may be appropriate for your older child.

Become an expert on financial assistance programs and your family's insurance benefits. Consider your life, health, and disability coverage when you move or change jobs. Cerebral palsy may be considered a preexisting condition and not be covered by a new insurance policy. Make sure major pieces of equipment like wheelchairs are added to your homeowner's or renter's insurance policies. This often protects the equipment in the case of theft or damage.

When possible, put some money aside for emergencies, necessary expenses, or vacations. Use an account that you can access easily like bank savings accounts or money market funds.

If you expect to have a certain amount of medical expenses during the year, look into flexible spending accounts through your employer or medical savings accounts through an insurance company. The money put into these accounts is not taxed, which can save you money. However, you must use the money you put into a flexible spending account by the end of the year or you lose it, and medical savings accounts require a large out-of-pocket deductible.

Refer to the United States Internal Revenue Service (IRS) manual on child and dependent care to learn what tax exemptions apply to you. In addition to medical bills, other expenses might be tax deductible. Those related to modifying your home for wheelchair access, transportation to appointments, or programs prescribed by your child's doctor are a few examples.

Consider starting a *special needs trust* for your child. First, get a tax identification number from the IRS. A special needs trust can manage your child's money without risking his eligibility for government benefits. These trusts are particularly useful for adults with cerebral palsy who live semi-independently. Learn how deposits and withdrawals affect the trust. Taking money out of the trust and giving it to your child as spending money may count as unearned income. If this puts him over his income limit, his Supplemental Security Income or Medicaid benefits will be reduced or lost for the month. A certified financial planner can teach you to use the trust successfully.

Parents need to write a legal will. When you decide how your estate will be divided, keep your child's government funding in mind. Direct inheritances or benefits from your insurance policies, retirement, or pension funds can be taken away if your child receives disability benefits. Instead, the inheritance or benefits could be placed in a trust fund. Consult a lawyer who understands disability laws and programs when you plan your estate.

Include all of your family members in these major decisions. Make sure that the family comes to a decision about who will care for a child with cerebral palsy after the parents pass away. Perhaps a grandparent, sibling, uncle, or close family friend will assume this responsibility. Let appropriate people know where important documents are kept. Include social, medical, and financial listings and contacts in your child's care notebook.

If your child with cerebral palsy will always need supervision or total care to maintain his health and safety, you need to apply for *guardianship*. Parents of an adult with a disability are not automatically made legal guardian. Guardianship is a legal process that determines a person's competence or ability to take care of himself. Full guardianship will be needed if a person depends on others for all caretaking. Limited guardianship is an option for people who can live mostly on their own but need help making decisions about medical care or managing money. Both parents can be named as coguardians. Others can also apply for guardianship or coguardianship. You need to start the process of applying for guardianship before your child's twenty-first birthday. If you fail to apply for guardianship, you may lose the right to make medical and financial decisions for your adult child with cerebral palsy. If the family does not name a guardian, the child may become a ward of the state.

Last but not least important, parents should involve their child with a disability in financial planning. An essential way to prepare your child for his financial future is to begin teaching money skills at an early age. As he learns to count, your child can learn the differences between coins and bills and what they can buy. Through chores or rewards, he can save money and then learn how to spend it wisely. By teaching your child money management skills, you begin to give him financial planning abilities that will last a lifetime. Your child with cerebral palsy should be involved in family meetings regarding finances. As much as possible, he should take part in decision making. After all, you and your family are planning together for his successful financial future.

# 55

# LETTING GO

The most important responsibility for any parent is to raise a child and help the child reach her greatest level of independence. The ultimate goal is for the child to feel that her life is purposeful and meaningful. A young adult should feel confident that she can make her own way in the world with less protection from her parents.

Very early on, parents must begin to *let go*. Letting go is hundreds of tiny actions that build on each other. They give your child the confidence to say one day, "Look Mommy, I can do it all by myself." Letting go begins as early as allowing your child to lie on her tummy on the floor while she masters holding up her head or scooting toward her favorite toy. Resist the urge to pick your child up immediately and rescue her when she cries. Letting go is as simple as waiting to give your child her juice until she points to her cup. It means waking your child thirty minutes early so she can struggle to put her own shirt on before the school bus arrives. Letting go is teaching your child to get up when she falls and pick up those crutches again. It means finding a great baby-sitter or respite program so you can take a vacation with your spouse. Letting go is allowing your teenager with cerebral palsy to participate in a vocational training program with a job coach. It means being supportive when she begins to date a young man that she met at a local rehabilitation center or at school.

Parents need to have a life beyond raising their children. Even when their child is severely disabled, parents usually cannot meet all of their child's needs forever. Most children with cerebral palsy will grow to adulthood and will outlive their parents. Unfortunately, some children with cerebral palsy will not live longer than their parents. In times of such loss, parents will need to grieve and then also let go.

Many parents become overwhelmed when looking for work, a place to live, or attendant care for a young adult with cerebral palsy. Parents tell themselves, "It's too hard. There aren't enough programs. The waiting lists are too long. My child's disabilities are too severe. My child's medical problems are too great. It's too expensive."

Parents can live in denial, convinced they will be able to care for their child forever, causing their child to miss the opportunity to grow and mature. Parents with firm intentions to keep their child at home forever sometimes become ill, die, or acquire disabilities themselves. These may make caring for an adult with cerebral palsy in the home impossible.

Throughout the child's life, parents need to investigate resources and build a network for this future adult that includes housing, transportation, medical care, financial support, supported employment, useful activity, attendant care, and access to family and friends. Helping your child have a more independent life and working to build a successful network is a greater gift of love for your child than trying desperately to do it all yourself. Do not expect your other adult children to assume the burden of care for their brother or sister with cerebral palsy. Look for a wide variety of options. Include an option of living in the community with family nearby so that you can let go and still have frequent contact.

Know what programs exist in your local area, your city, your state, and at the national level that might help your child. If you are uncertain, look for a case manager who can help you. Enlist expert legal and financial advice early to help you plan ahead.

Through preparation, you and your child will be ready for the next step in life. The most loving gift parents can give is to plan ahead to help their child have the most active, independent life possible and then lovingly *let go* into full participation in the wider world. Raising a child with cerebral palsy is indeed a unique and special journey.

# QUESTIONS AND ANSWERS

**Should my child with cerebral palsy take adapted physical education, regular P.E., or be excused from gym?**

It is important for your child to have regular physical exercise. Some children with mild cerebral palsy enjoy regular P.E. class. Other children use adapted P.E. to practice individual skills such as weight lifting, to prepare for Special Olympics, to do stretching, or to practice driving a power wheelchair. Some children prefer to take a karate or dance class away from school.

**My child doesn't want to wear his braces or splints. Should I force him to?**

If it prevents pain, muscle shortening, or damage to joints or if it greatly improves your child's ability to use a limb, wearing the brace or splint is important. Often, you can negotiate for him to wear it at certain times and take it off at other times. Long pants, high-topped shoes, or long sleeves can camouflage braces and splints.

**Sometimes when I move my child's hand or foot, it shakes rhythmically. What is this and does it hurt?**

This rhythmic shaking is called *clonus*. It is a response to a muscle being suddenly stretched. Clonus is often seen in children and adults with spastic cerebral palsy and is painless.

## QUESTIONS AND ANSWERS

**My therapist says my child needs a wheelchair. I'm afraid if I get her one she'll never learn to walk. What should I do?**

Many children with cerebral palsy walk for short distances and use a wheelchair for longer distances. It is important to give your child plenty of practice doing both. A wheelchair allows children to keep up with their friends and experience a wider world.

**My child's school has stopped giving him therapy. I think he still needs it. Can I force the school to give him therapy?**

Your child's public school is legally required only to provide therapy that directly supports his educational goals. Sometimes an advocate can help you work this out. Please see Keys 34 and 38 for more details.

**It seems easier to feed my child if I tip his head back. Is this safe?**

Tipping your child's head back for feeding is very dangerous. It opens the windpipe, possibly allowing food and liquid to enter the lungs. This can lead to choking, pneumonia, or even death. Consult your doctor or therapist for help.

**What is a swallow study?**

It is a special moving X-ray picture taken while your child is swallowing food or liquid. It helps determine if your child is chewing and swallowing safely. It shows if any food or liquid goes through the windpipe and into the lungs.

# GLOSSARY

**Action plan** an organized plan for solving a problem when encountered. It includes a time frame and assigns responsibility.

**Advocacy** to persuade and encourage other people, organizations, or governments to act in the best interest and protect the legal rights of a person or group such as children with cerebral palsy.

**Alignment** the straight, normal position of a body part.

**Apnea** a period of not breathing.

**Aspiration** inhaling/swallowing food or liquid into the lungs.

**Assistive technology** equipment that helps a person with a disability to perform tasks that would otherwise be very difficult or impossible.

**Ataxia** abnormal muscle tone characterized by unsteadiness, tremors, and staggering.

**Athetoid/Athetosis** abnormal muscle tone characterized by frequent sudden changes. It ranges from very limp to very stiff.

**Augmentative and alternative communication (AAC)** other simple or complicated forms of communication used by people who cannot speak effectively.

**Botulinum toxin** a medicine used to reduce spasticity temporarily by direct injection into a muscle or muscles.

**Bronchopulmonary dysplasia (BPD)** a chronic respiratory disorder usually occurring in children who have used breathing machines for a long time or were born prematurely.

**Case manager** a person who oversees, coordinates, and organizes a child's complete medical and/or educational program and assists with obtaining funding, authorizing treatment, and finding resources and equipment.

# GLOSSARY

**Cognition** another word for intelligence; describes what one knows and/or understands.

**Community integration** living within typical neighborhoods using local services and participating in community-based activities.

**Contractures** a degree of tightness in the muscles around a joint that limits joint movement.

**CT scan** computerized axial tomography, *cat* scan, is a specialized type of X ray that takes many cross-sectional pictures, producing a computer-generated image.

**Developmental** pertains to the process of a child maturing and learning new skills.

**Dislocation** occurs when a bone comes completely out of a joint. Requires intervention to be reconnected.

**Due process** legal rights and practices that ensure fair treatment regardless of disability. Commonly referred to in education settings.

**Early intervention** a free program that provides services to children zero to three years old who are at risk of or have been diagnosed with a disability.

**Electrical stimulation** treating a person with a small amount of electrical current to improve body function. Intended to relax, strengthen, and coordinate muscles.

**Electroencephalogram (EEG)** a test to measure electrical activity in the brain.

**Electromyography (EMG)** a test to measure electrical activity in muscles.

**Expressive language** the part of communication that includes forming and sharing information.

**504 Plan** a training plan for children who need support in order to participate equally in regular education.

**Food texture** the coarseness or fineness of a food.

**Function** a person's ability to do things that are essential for everyday life.

**Fundoplication (fundo)**  a surgical procedure that narrows the opening between the stomach and esophagus to decrease reflux.

**Gastroesophageal reflux**  a disorder that causes food in the stomach to return up through the esophagus.

**Gastrostomy tube (G-tube)**  a tube placed into part of the stomach for nutrition when eating by mouth is not possible or safe.

**Genetic**  a characteristic passed from parents to their children.

**Guardianship**  legal right to assume responsibility for another person's safety, health, and overall welfare.

**Habilitation**  helping someone with a disability learn skills for the first time so the person can function more independently.

**Hereditary**  see *Genetic*.

**Hydrocephalus**  excess fluid in the brain.

**Hypertonia**  high (tight or stiff) muscle tone.

**Hypotonia**  low (floppy or limp) muscle tone.

**Inclusion**  the process of integrating or including a child with special needs into a regular school program.

**Individualized education program (IEP)**  a specific written training plan used in school for special education.

**Individualized family services plan (IFSP)**  a specific written training plan used in early intervention.

**Individualized habilitation plan (IHP)**  a specific written training plan used in residential settings or when habilitation training is provided in a person's home.

**Inhibitory casting**  encasing a body part in plaster or fiberglass in a controlled position to relax tight muscle tone.

**Interdisciplinary team**  a combination of different types of professionals who evaluate and work with a child separately or together and share ideas for individual and combined programs.

**Kyphosis**  a forward curvature of the spine usually in the upper back and shoulder area in a *C* or hump shape.

**Least restrictive environment**  an educational setting as similar to same age peers as possible.

# GLOSSARY

**Magnetic resonance imaging (MRI)** a special type of test that uses a magnet to show detailed pictures of body parts. Similar to CT scan.

**Mainstreaming** see *Inclusion*.

**Mediation** using an impartial person to hear disputes between parents and school systems to come to a peaceful resolution.

**Mental retardation** below normal intelligence with impairments in life skills.

**Milestones** typical steps children achieve as they grow and develop.

**Multidisciplinary team** a combination of different types of professionals who evaluate and work with a child separately and meet as a team to discuss their separate findings and goals.

**Muscle tone** the amount of tightness or floppiness in muscles, which affects coordinated movement.

**Network** an informal or formal way to gain information and build a support system.

**Neurodevelopmental treatment (NDT)** a specialized therapy approach that encourages normal movement and discourages abnormal reflexes, postures, and movements. Requires certification.

**Neurology** the study of the nervous system, which consists of the brain, spinal cord, and nerves.

**Nutrition** provides foods and liquids for healthy brain and body growth.

**Orthopedics** a medical specialty focused on disorders of the muscles, joints, and bones.

**Orthotics/Orthosis** splints or braces made of hard plastic and/or metal.

**Orthotist** a person who specializes in fitting and making orthotics.

**Osteotomy** a surgical procedure that corrects the alignment of a bone.

**Physical medicine and rehabilitation** a specialized area of medicine focused on helping people become as independent as possible and returning them to a more normal lifestyle.

**Positioning** using pillows or adaptive equipment to achieve better body alignment, function, and comfort.

**Psychosocial** relates to a child's mental and emotional needs and development.

**Puree** foods blended to a yogurt-like consistency.

**Receptive language** the part of communication that includes gaining and understanding information.

**Reflex** an automatic movement, one not under voluntary control.

**Rehabilitation** to restore a person to an earlier state of independent function.

**Related services** services necessary to participate in education.

**Resource** information, program, or service that might benefit your child and family.

**Rhizotomy** an extensive neurological surgery to reduce spasticity permanently.

**Scoliosis** a curvature of the spine to the side, usually in a $C$ or $S$ shape.

**Seizures** abnormal electrical activity in the brain.

**Sensory integration (SI)** a specialized therapy approach that addresses the way the brain processes information from the senses and their impact on movement, learning, and behavior. Requires certification.

**Serial casting** casting a body part with limited movement and replacing the cast periodically to increase the amount of movement.

**Spasticity** an abnormal increase or tightness in muscle tone.

**Splint** lightweight positioning device usually for the hand or foot.

**Static encephalopathy** a general abnormal functioning of the brain that does not worsen as the child grows older. Often used as another name for cerebral palsy.

**Strabismus** crossed eyes, failure of both eyes to focus on the same object, usually as a result of eye-muscle imbalance.

**Subluxation** a partial dislocation; the bone is loose in a joint but can slide back in the socket through manipulation or by itself.

**Switches**  a homemade or manufactured device to activate or use battery-operated and electronic devices.

**Tenotomy**  a surgical procedure for a contracture that lengthens the tendon attaching the muscle to the bone.

**Tracheostomy**  a surgical opening in the neck that connects to the trachea (main breathing tube).

**Transdisciplinary team**  a combination of different types of professionals who train one another so that any member can address most of a child's needs. Consultation is used when more expertise is required.

**Transition**  the process of changing and moving from one thing to another, as with moving from high school to adulthood.

**Ventilator (respirator)**  a machine used to help a person breathe.

# TIPS FOR POSITIONING YOUR CHILD

1. Ask your child's physical and occupational therapists for ideas to meet your child's specific positioning needs.
2. Find a balance between a position that maintains body alignment and one that allows your child some freedom to move comfortably.
3. As much as possible, position your child so that his body is in a straight line and both sides look the same.
4. Pillows, towel rolls, small beanbags, and stuffed animals make good positioning tools.
5. In addition to providing a way to prevent deformity, stretch muscles, and protect the skin, positioning can help your child do an activity better. Use good positioning when he is eating, bathing, playing, watching TV, doing homework, and so on.

**Supine—Lying on back**
    a. Place his trunk in a straight position.
    b. Keep his legs from rolling out into a "frog" position or crossing into a "scissor" position.
    c. Keep your child's legs from always rolling to one side.
    d. Keep his head from extending backward.

**Prone—Lying on abdomen**
    a. Place your child's trunk in a straight position.
    b. Keep his legs from rolling to one side.
    c. Place your child's arms and head in a comfortable position.

d. To work on holding his head up and using his arms, place a pillow or wedge under your child's chest and let him rest on his forearms.

**Side-lying—Lying on right or left side**
   a. His head and trunk should be aligned.
   b. Rest your child's back against a firm flat surface if his posture tends to be rounded forward.
   c. Bend his top leg.
   d. Place a pillow between his knees.
   e. Encourage arm and hand movements with a toy. Your child may be able to play better in side-lying than other positions.

**Sitting**
   a. Discourage "W" sitting, where the inside surface of your child's legs is on the floor letting his legs form the letter *W*.
   b. Use a firm surface for support.
   c. Help your child sit up straight and with good posture. Use extra supports as needed to prevent him from slumping forward or to the side.
   d. Make sure his hips are all the way back on the seat when using any type of chair. Use a snug lap belt to maintain this position.

Various types of homemade and manufactured equipment can be used for positioning. These include wedges, side lyers, corner chairs, feeder seats, wheelchairs, standing frames, and many more. Ask your child's therapists for instructions and recommendations.

# SUGGESTED READING

**Personalized**

Mathews, R. *Baby Book: For the Developmentally Challenged Child.* Contact *Exceptional Parent* (see Magazines and Newsletters), Exceptional Parent Library (a baby book specially designed for children with disabilities).

**General**

Baker, B.L. and Brightman, A.J. *Steps to Independence: A Skills Training Guide for Parents and Teachers of Children with Special Needs,* 2nd edition. Baltimore, MD: Paul H. Brookes, 1989.

Binstock, C. *After the Diagnosis: A Practical Guide for Families Raising Children with Disabilities.* Manassis, VA: E.M. Press, 1997.

Callanan, C.R. *Since Owen: A Parent to Parent Guide for Care of the Disabled Child.* Baltimore, MD: John Hopkins University Press, 1990.

Featherstone, H. *A Difference in the Family: Life with a Disabled Child.* New York: Basic Books, 1980.

Finnie, N.R. *Handling the Young Cerebral Palsied Child at Home,* 2nd edition. New York: Penguin Books, USA, 1975 (may be available free by request from your local United Cerebral Palsy Association [UCPA]).

French, C. Gonzalez, R.T., and Tronson-Simpson, J. *Caring for People with Multiple Disabilities: An Interdisciplinary Guide for Caregivers.* Tucson, AZ: Therapy Skill Builders, 1991.

Geralis, E., ed. *Children with Cerebral Palsy: A Parent's Guide.* Bethesda, MD: Woodbine House, 1981.

## SUGGESTED READING

McAnaney, K.D. *I Wish: Dreams and Realities of Parenting a Special Needs Child*. Sacramento, CA: United Cerebral Palsy Association, 1992.

Miller, F. and Bach, S. *Cerebral Palsy: A Complete Guide for Caregiving*. Contact *Exceptional Parent* (see Magazines and Newsletters), Exceptional Parent Library.

Morris, L.R. and Schulz, L. *Creative Play Activities for Children with Disabilities: A Resource Book for Teachers and Parents*, 2nd ed. Champaign, IL: Human Kinetics, 1989.

Russell, L.M. et al. *Planning for the Future: Providing a Meaningful Life for a Child with Disability After Your Death*. Contact *Exceptional Parent* (see Magazines and Newsletters), Exceptional Parent Library.

Russell, L.M. and Grant, A.E. *The Life Planning Workbook*. Contact *Exceptional Parent*, (see Magazines and Newsletters), Exceptional Parent Library.

Weiss, S. *Each of Us Remembers: Parents of Children with Cerebral Palsy Answer Your Questions*. Washington, D.C.: United Cerebral Palsy Association, 1993.

### Family

Klein, S.D. and Schleifer, M.J., ed. *It Isn't Fair: Siblings of Children with Disabilities*. Contact *Exceptional Parent* (see Magazines and Newsletters), Exceptional Parent Library.

Lobato, D.J. *Brothers, Sisters and Special Needs: Information and Activities for Helping Young Siblings of Children with Chronic Illnesses and Developmental Disabilities*. Baltimore, MD: Paul H. Brookes, 1990.

Meyer, D.J., Vadasy, P.F., and Fewell, R.R. *Living with a Brother or Sister with Special Needs: A Book for Siblings*. Seattle, WA: University of Washington Press, 1985.

Pinkava, M.J. *A Handful of Hope: Helpful Suggestions for Grandparents of Children with Disabilities*. Phoenix, AZ: Pilot Parent Partnerships, 1991.

Thompson, M. *My Brother Matthew*. Rockville, MD: Woodbine Press, 1992 (intended for preschool age siblings).

## Children's books written for and about children with disabilities and their friends

Exley, H. *What It's Like to Be Me*, 2nd ed. New York: Friendship Press, 1984.

Turtlebooks, Jason and Nordic Publishers, P.O. Box 441, Holidaysburg, PA 16648, (814) 696-2920.

### Nonfiction

Killilea, M. *Karen*. New York: Prentice Hall, 1952. (a mother of a daughter with cerebral palsy tells her family's story of coping with Karen's struggles and triumphs of growing up in the 1950s).

Killilea, M. *With Love From Karen*. New York: Dell Publishers, 1963. (a sequel to *Karen* that follows Karen's journey into young adulthood).

Smith, M. *Growing Up with Cerebral Palsy*, Waco, TX: W. R. S. Publishing, 1995. (Out of print but available through author: (510) 228-8928.)

### Magazines and Newsletters

*Accent on Living*. Cheever Publishing, P.O. Box 700, Bloomington, IL 61702, (800) 787-8444 (provides information on daily living with personal experiences from people with disabilities).

*Exceptional Parent*. Customer Service, P.O. Box 3000, Department EP, Denville, NJ 07834, (800) 247-8080. Exceptional Parent Library (800) 535-1910.

*Mainstream*. 2973 Beech Street, San Diego, CA 92102, (619) 234-3138 (provides information on a wide variety of topics affecting people with disabilities).

*NICHCY News Digest*. National Information Center for Children and Youth with Disabilities, P.O. Box 1492, Washington, D.C. 20013, (800) 999-5599.

*Peoplenet*. P.O. Box 897, Levittown, NY 11756, (516) 579-4043 (provides information by and for people with disabilities about relationships and sexuality).

*Professional Parent Magazine*. Arduous Publication, P.O. Box 820813, Houston, TX 77282-0813, (713) 467-5555 (provides information for parents of children in special education).

## SUGGESTED READING

*Teaching Exceptional Children.* Council for Exceptional Children, 1920 Association Drive, Reston, VA 20191, (703) 620-3660 (special education news and latest teaching strategies).

*Team Rehab Reports: For Professionals in Rehabilitation Technology and Services.* P.O. Box 16778, North Hollywood, CA 91615-6778, (800) 543-4116 (provides information about assistive technology, rehabilitation, and recreation).

# RESOURCES

Key:  +  referral/information
      o  local programs
      x  newsletter/publications
      =  funding/service source

**Cerebral Palsy and Related Conditions**
National Brain Injury Association
1776 Massachusetts Avenue, N.W., Suite 100
Washington, D.C. 20036
(800) 444-6443 +

National Organization on Rare Disorders (NORD)
100 Route 37
P.O. Box 8923
New Fairfield, CT 06812-8923
(800) 999-6673 +

The Arc (formerly the Association for Retarded Citizens of the U.S.)
500 E. Border Street, Suite 300
Arlington, TX 76010
(800) 433-5255 + o

United Cerebral Palsy Association (UCPA)
1660 L Street, N.W., Suite 700
Washington, D.C. 20036
(800) USA-5UCP + o =

**General Disabilities and Information**
Association for the Care of Children's Health (ACCH)
7910 Woodmont Avenue, #300
Bethesda, MD 20814
(800) 808-2224 + x

Clearinghouse on Disability Information
Office of Special Education and Rehabilitative Services (OSERS)
330 C Street, S.W., Room 3132, Switzer Building
Washington, D.C. 20202-2524
(202) 205-8241 + x

Collaboration Among Parents and Health Care Professionals (CAPP): National Parent Resource Center
Federation for Children with Special Needs
95 Berkeley Street, Suite 104
Boston, MA 02116
(800) 331-0688 x

National Information Center for Children and Youth with Disabilities (NICHCY)
P.O. Box 1492
Washington, D.C. 20013-1492
(800) 695-0285 + x

National Information Clearinghouse (NIC) for Infants with Disabilities and Life-Threatening Conditions
Center for Developmental Disabilities
University of South Carolina
Columbia, SC 29208
(800) 922-9234, extension 201 +

National Rehabilitation Information Center (NARIC)
8455 Colesville Road, Suite 935
Silver Spring, MD 20910-3319
(800) 346-2742 + x

Technical Assistance for Parent Programs (TAPP)
Federation for Children with Special Needs
95 Berkeley Street, Suite 104
Boston, MA 02116
(800) 331-0688 x

**Organizations and Health Care**
March of Dimes Birth Defects Foundation
1275 Mamaroneck Avenue
White Plains, NY 10605
(914) 428-7100
(888) MO-DIMES + o =
(pregnancy and birth defects information)

National Easter Seal Society
230 West Monroe Street
Chicago, IL 60606
(800) 221-6827 + o =

Scottish Rite Centers
1733 Sixteenth Street, N.W.
Washington, D.C. 20009-3199
(800) 776-2766 + =

Shriner's Hospitals for Crippled Children
2900 Rocky Point Drive
Tampa, FL 33607
(800) 237-5055 + o =

United Way of America
701 North Fairfax Street
Alexandria, VA 22314-2045
(703) 836-7100 + o =

**Financial Assistance**
Disabled Children's Relief Fund (DCRF)
402 Pennsylvania Avenue
Freeport, NY 11520
(516) 377-1605 (leave message for return call) + =

Foundation Center
79 Fifth Avenue
New York, NY 10003-3076
(212) 620-4230 + x
(grants)

Internal Revenue Service
Consumer Information Center
Department 92
Pueblo, CO 81009
(800) 829-1040 + x

National Foundation for
 Consumer Credit
8611 Second Avenue, Suite 100
Silver Spring, MD 20910
(800) 388-2227 + o
(money management and
 budgeting)

Social Security Administration
Department of Health and
 Human Services
6401 Security Boulevard
Baltimore, MD 21235
(800) 772-1605 + =

**Family Organizations**
American Association of
 Retired Person (AARP)
Grandparent Information
 Center
601 E Street, N.W.
Washington, D.C. 20049
(202) 434-2296 + o x
(grandparents raising
 grandchildren)

DIRECT LINK for the Disabled,
 Inc.
P.O. Box 1036
Solvang, CA 93464
(805) 688-1603 + x

Mothers United for Moral
 Support (MUMS)
National Parent-to-Parent
 Network
150 Custer Court
Green Bay, WI 54301-1243
(414) 336-5333 (leave message
 for return call) + x

National Father's Network
Kinderling Center
16120 N.E. 8th Street
Bellevue, WA 98008-3937
(206) 747-4004 + x

National Foster Parent
 Association (NFPA)
9 Dartmoor Drive
Crystal Lake, IL 60014
(815) 455-2527 + o x

Parents Helping Parents
The Parent-Directed Family
 Resource Center for Children
 with Special Needs
3041 Olcott Street
Santa Clara, CA 95054
(408) 727-5775 + x

The Sibling Support Project
Children's Hospital and Medical
    Center
P.O. Box 5371, CL-09
Seattle, WA 98105-0371
(206) 368-4911 + o x

**Advocacy and Legal Rights**
Disability Rights Education and
    Defense Fund (DREDF)
2212 Sixth Street
Berkeley, CA 94710
(510)644-2555 + x

National Association of
    Protection and Advocacy
    Systems (NAPAS)
900 Second Street, N.E.
Suite 211
Washington, D.C. 20002
(202) 408-9514 + o x

People First International
P.O. Box 12642
Salem, OR 97309
(503) 362-0336 + o
(leave message for return call)
(self-advocacy, leadership
    skills)

**Early Intervention**
Brazelton Center for Mental
    Health
(formerly LINKS)
1101 Fifteenth Street, N.W.
Washington, D.C. 20005
(202) 467-5730 + x

Head Start Bureau
Administration on Children,
    Youth and Families
U.S. Department of Health and
    Human Services
P.O. Box 1182
Washington, D.C. 20013
(202) 205-8347 + o

**Education**
Americom Council on Rural
    Special Education (ACRES)
University of Utah
221 Milton Bennion Hall
Salt Lake City, UT 84112
(801) 585-5659 + o x

Council for Exceptional
    Children (CEC)
1920 Association Drive
Reston, VA 20191-1589
(703) 620-3660 + x

National Association of Private
    Schools for Exceptional
    Children (NAPSEC)
1522 K Street, N.W., Suite 1032
Washington, D.C. 20005
(202) 408-3338 + x

National Committee for Citizens
    in Education
900 2nd Street, N.E., Suite 8
Washington, D.C. 20002-3557
(202) 408-0447 + x
(National Coalition for Parent
    Involvement in Education—
    NCPIE—resource guide)

## Higher Education and Transition

American Association of University Affiliated Programs (UAP) for Persons with Developmental Disabilities
8630 Fenton Street, Suite 410
Silver Spring, MD 20910
(301) 588-8252 + x

Association on Higher Education and Disability (AHEAD)
P.O. Box 21192
Columbus, OH 43221-0192
(614) 488-4972 + x
(choosing colleges, support groups)

HEATH Resource Center
American Council on Education
One Dupont Circle, N.W.
Suite 800
Washington, D.C. 20036-1193
(202) 939-9320 + x

National Center for Youth with Disabilities (NCYD)
University of Minnesota
Box 721
420 Delaware Street, S.E.
Minneapolis, MN 55455
(612) 626-2825 + x

## Employment

Davis Memorial Goodwill Industries, Inc.
2200 South Dakota Avenue, N.E.
Washington, D.C. 20018
(202) 636-4225 + o

Electronics Industries Foundation
Project with Industry
2500 Wilson Boulevard
Arlington, VA 22201
(703) 907-7400 +

## Independent Living

Access/Abilities
P.O. Box 458
Mill Valley, CA 94942
(415) 388-3250 +

National Council on Independent Living
2111 Wilson Boulevard, Suite 405
Arlington, VA 22201
(703) 525-3406 +

## Respite Care and Home Care

ARCH National Resource Center for Crisis Nurseries and Respite Care Services
800 Eastowne Drive, Suite 105
Chapel Hill, NC 27514
(800) 473-1727 +

National Association for Homecare
228 7th Street, S.E.
Washington, D.C. 20003
(202) 547-7424 +

# RESOURCES

**Recreation**
Association for Theatre and Accessibility
National Arts and Disability Center
UCLA University Affiliated Program
3000 UCLA Medical Plaza
Room 3330
Los Angeles, CA 90095-6967
(310) 794-1141 +

Disabled Sports USA
451 Hungerford Drive #100
Rockville, MD 20850
(301) 217-0960 (leave message for return call) + o
(sports and recreation)

National Institute of Art and Disabilities (NIAD)
551 23rd Street
Richmond, CA 94804
(510) 620-0290 +
(creative visual arts)

National Lekotek Center
2100 Ridge Avenue
Evanston, IL 60201
(800) 366-PLAY + o
(toy lending libraries)

National Library Service for the Blind and Physically Handicapped
The Library of Congress
1291 Taylor Street, N.W.
Washington, D.C. 20542
(800) 424-8567 + x
(loans books in Braille and on tape, recreation resources)

Special Olympics International Office
1325 G Street, N.W., Suite 500
Washington, D.C. 20005
(202) 628-3630 o x

United States Cerebral Palsy Athletic Association
200 Harrison Avenue
Newport, RI 02840
(401) 848-2460 + o x
(competitive sports at local through international levels)

Winners on Wheels (WOW)
2842 Business Park Avenue
Fresno, CA 93727-3386
(800) WOW-TALK + o
(various recreational activities)

**Therapy**
American Occupational Therapy Association (AOTA)
4720 Montgomery Lane
P.O. Box 31220
Bethesda, MD 20824-1120
(800) 377-8555 +

American Physical Therapy
  Association (APTA)
1111 North Fairfax Street
Alexandria, VA 22314
(800) 999-2782 +

American Speech-Language-
  Hearing Association (ASHA)
10801 Rockville Pike
Rockville, MD 20852
(800) 638-8255 +

Delta Society
289 Perimeter Road East
Renton, WA 98055-1329
(800) 809-2714 + o x
(service animals, pet therapy,
  hippotherapy)

**Sex Issues**
Sex Information and Education
  Council of the United States
  (SIECUS)
130 W. 42nd Street, Suite 350
New York, NY 10036-7802
(212) 819-9770 + x

**Publishers**
Paul H. Brookes Publishing
  Company
P.O. Box 10624
Baltimore, MD 21285-9945
(800) 638-3775 x

Physiological Corporation
Communication and Therapy
  Skill Builders
555 Academic Court
San Antonio, TX 78204
(800) 220-0756 x

# ASSISTIVE TECHNOLOGY RESOURCES

Key:  AAC    augmentative and alternative communication devices
      ADL    activities of daily living equipment: bathing, dressing, grooming, writing, and so on
      Rehab  pediatric rehabilitation/therapy equipment
      WC     wheelchairs

**General Listings**
ABLE DATA
8455 Colesville Road, Suite 935
Silver Spring, MD 20910-3319
(800) 227-0216
(information on specific devices and classes of assistive technology)

Trace Resourcebook
Trace R&D Center
S-151 Waisman Center
1500 Highland Avenue
Madison, WI 53705
(608) 263-2309
(information on assistive technologies for communication, control, and computer access)

**Assistive Technology Organizations**
Rehabilitation Engineering and Assistive Technology Society of North America (RESNA)
1700 N. Moore Street, Suite 1540
Arlington, VA 22209
(703) 524-6686
(provides international conferences, technical assistance, and referrals for recycled equipment)

TASH, Inc.
91 Station Street, Unit 1
Ajax, ON L1S 3H2
Canada
(800) 463-5685

(provides conferences, technical assistance, and a source for adapted switches and computer modifications)

**Manufacturers and Suppliers**

RG Abernathy, Inc.
P.O. Box 11733
Winston-Salem, NC 27116
(800) 334-0128
(custom orthopedic shoes)

AbleNet, Inc.
1081 10th Avenue, S.E.
Minneapolis, MN 55414
(800) 322-0956
(adapted switches, AAC)

Achievement Products, Inc.
P.O. Box 9033
Canton, OH 44711
(800) 373-4699
(rehab)

Acor Orthopaedic, Inc.
18530 S. Miles Parkway
Cleveland, OH 44218
(800) 237-2267
(custom orthotics)

Barrier Free Lifts, Inc.
9230 Prince William Street
Manassas, VA 22110
(800) 582-8732
(ceiling-mounted and floor model lifts)

Burkhart, Linda J.
6201 Candle Court
Eldersburge, MD 21784
(410) 795-4561
(adapted switches, homemade switch instruction manuals)

Cascade Prosthetics and Orthotics, Inc.
134 Pince Avenue
Bellingham, WA 98226
(800) 848-7332
(custom orthotics)

Clarke Health Care Products, Inc.
PIIP-ICM Bldg
1003 International Drive
Oakdale, PA 15071-9223
(412) 695-2122
(bathlifts)

Columbus McKinnon Corp.
Mobility Products Division
140 John James Audubon Parkway
Amherst, NY 14228-1197
(800) 888-0985
(lift and transfer systems)

Comfort House
189 Frelinghuysen Avenue
Newark, NJ 07114
(201) 242-8080
(ADL)

Convaid Products, Inc.
3541-A Lomita Boulevard
Torrance, CA 90505
(800) 552-1020
(strollers)

## ASSISTIVE TECHNOLOGY RESOURCES

Creative Switch Industries
P.O. Box 5256
Des Moines, IA 50306
(515) 287-5748
(adapted switches)

Danmar Products, Inc.
221 Jackson Industrial Drive
Ann Arbor, MI 48103
(800) 783-1998
(helmets, pool equipment, ADL)

Don Johnston Incorporated
P.O. Box 639
1000 N. Rand Road, Building 115
Wauconda, IL 60084
(800) 999-4660
(adapted switches, computer software)

Edmark Corporation
6727 185th Avenue, N.E.
P.O. Box 97021
Redmond, WA 98073-9721
(computer software, *catalog)

Electric Mobility Corporation
1 Mobility Plaza
Sewell, NJ 08080
(800) 662-4548
(power scooters, WC)

Equipment Shop
P.O. Box 33
Bedford, MA 01730
(800) 525-7681
(rehab, positioning)

E-Z Company USA LLC
P.O. Box 13
Columbus, KS 66725
(800) 492-3279
(ADL)

E-Z ON Products, Inc. of Florida
500 Commerce Way W
Jupiter, FL 33458
(800) 323-6598
(secure vests and belts for transportation)

Flaghouse, Inc.
601 Flaghouse Drive
Hasbrouck Heights, NJ 07604-3116
(800) 793-7900
(rehab, ADL, *catalog)

Freedom Designs, Inc.
2241 Madera Road
Simi Valley, CA 93065
(800) 331-8551
(custom seating systems, WC)

Guardian Products
4175 Guardian Street
Simi Valley, CA 93063
(800) 423-8034
(walking aids, ADL)

Guildcraft, Inc.
100 Fire Tower Drive
Tonawanda, NY 14150
(716) 743-8336
(therapeutic craft activities)

Invacare
899 Cleveland Street
Elyria, OH 44035
(800) 333-6900
(WC, ADL)

Jay Medical, Ltd.
4745 Walnut Street
Boulder, CO 80301
(800) 648-8282
(seating for WC)

Jesana, Ltd.
979 Saw Mill River Road
Yonkers, NY 10710
(800) 443-4728
(AAC, rehab, adaptive toys, sensory stimulation, *catalog)

Kaye Products, Inc.
535 Dimmocks Mill Road
Hillsborough, NC 27278
(919) 732-6444
(walking aids, recreation)

Kid-Kart, Inc.
732 Cruiser Lane
Belgrade, MT 59714
(800) 388-5278
(strollers)

Kuschall of America
708 Via Alondra
Camarillo, CA 93012-8713
(800) 654-4768
(WC)

Lift Aid, Inc.
38281 Schoolcraft Road, Suite B
Livonia, MI 48150
(313) 432-9500
(overhead lifts)

Maddak, Inc.
6 Industrial Road
Pequannock, NJ 07440
(800) 443-4926
(ADL, recreation)

Merry Walker Corporation
P.O. Box 9
9804 Main Street
Hebron, IL 60034
(815) 648-4125
(walking aids)

Mulholland Positioning Systems, Inc.
P.O. Box 391
215 N. 12th Street
Santa Paula, CA 93061
(800) 543-4769
(standers, WC)

North Coast Medical, Inc.
187 Stauffer Boulevard
San Jose, CA 95125-1042
(800) 821-9319
(ADL)

Ortho-Kinetics, Inc.
W220 N507 Springdale Road
P.O. Box 1647
Waukesha, WI 53187-1647
(800) 824-1068
(standers, WC)

## ASSISTIVE TECHNOLOGY RESOURCES

Parrot Software
6505 Pleasant Lake Court
West Bloomfield, MI 48322
(800) 727-7681
(computer software)

Plum Enterprises, Inc.
P.O. Box 283
Worcester, PA 19490
(800) 321-PLUM
(helmets)

Prentke Romich Company
1022 Heyl Road
Wooster, OH 44691
(800) 262-1933
(AAC, computer modifications, environmental controls)

Prime Engineering
4838 W. Jacquelyn, #105
Fresno, CA 93722
(800) 82S-TAND
(standing frames)

Quickie Designs
2842 Business Park Avenue
Fresno, CA 93727
(800) 456-8168
(WC, seating)

Rifton Equipment
Rt. 213, Box 901
Rifton, NY 12471
(800) 374-3866
(positioning, standers, walking aids)

Sabel Shoe Company
P.O. Box 644
Jenkintown, PA 19046
(215) 885-1772
(orthopedic shoes)

Sammons Preston, Inc.
4 Sammons Court
Bolingbrook, IL 60440
(800) 323-5547
(rehab, ADL, *catalog)

Sentient Systems Technology, Inc.
2100 Wharton Street, Suite 630
Pittsburgh, PA 15203
(800) 344-1778
(AAC)

Smith & Nephew Rolyan, Inc.
One Quality Drive
P.O. Box 1005
Germantown, WI 53022
(800) 558-8633
(ADL)

Snug Seat, Inc.
10810 Independence Pointe Parkway
Matthews, NC 28106
(800) 336-7684
(strollers, car seats, standers)

TherAdapt Products, Inc.
17 W. 163 Oak Lane
Bensenville, Il 60106
(800) 261-4919
(rehab, positioning)

KEYS TO PARENTING A CHILD WITH CEREBRAL PALSY

Tip Top Mobility, Inc.
101 E. Central Avenue
P.O. Box 5009
Minot, ND 58702-5009
(800) 735-5958
(cartop WC lift)

Toys for Special Children, Inc.
385 Warburton Avenue
Hastings-on-Hudson, NY 10706
(800) 832-8697
(adapted switches and toys)

TRIAID, Inc.
P.O. Box 1364
Cumberland, MD 21502
(800) 306-6777
(adapted switches)

Tumble Forms
4 Sammons Court
Boling Brook, IL 60440
(800) 323-5547
(positioning, standers)

Unishape Adaptive Positioning
    Equipment
1630 30th Street, Suite 202
Boulder, CO 80304
(303) 443-8348
(positioning)

Wayne County Regional
    Education Service Agency
ADAMLAB
33500 Van Born Rd
Wayne, MI 48184
(313) 467-1415
(AAC)

Worldwide Engineering
3240 N. Delaware Street
Chandler, AZ 85225-1100
(800) 848-3433
(car carriers for WC and
    scooters)

Zygo Industries, Inc.
P.O. Box 1008
Portland, OR 97207
(800) 234-6006
(AAC, adapted switches)

# INDEX

Abilities, 15
Acceptance, 22
Accessibility, 142
Accidents, 7
Action plan, 152
Activities of daily living, 64, 80
Adaptive toys, 96–98, 140–141
Adolescents, 67, 166
Adolescent siblings, 40
Adult day care, 161
Adult services, 158
Agenesis of corpus collosum, 6
Alertness, 4
Americans with Disabilities Act, 46, 159
Anger, 21
Animals, 146
Apnea, 70
Art therapy, 81
Aspiration, 70, 75
Assistive technology, 96, 140–143
    resources list for, 205–210
Associations, 178
Athetoid cerebral palsy, 8–9
Augmentative or alternative communication devices, 138–139, 142
Awakeness, 4

Babies, 2
    calming, awakeness, alertness problems of, 4
    feeding problems of, 3
    movement problems of, 3
Baby sitter, 94
Baclofen pump, 83
Bargaining, 21
Behavior, 4
Behavior management, 104–107

Biofeedback, 85–86
Birth control, 167, 169
Bladder training program, 78
Bleeding, 6
Blood vessel abnormalities, 6
Body positioning, 100, 136, 192–193
Bones, 58
Books, list of, 194–196
Botulinum toxin, 83–84
Braces, 85, 184
Brain damage, 5
Brain structures, undeveloped, 6
Breathing problems, 70
Bronchopulmonary dysplasia, 70
Brothers, 37–41

Calmness, 4
Care notebook, 92–93
Carl D. Perkins Vocational and Applied Technology Education Act, 159
Carrying, 50
Case manager, 79, 118, 175–176
Casts, 84
Celebrating small accomplishments, 32
Cerebral palsy
    ataxic type, 9
    athetoid type, 8–9
    babies with, 2–4
    causes of, 6–7
    defined, 5
    hypotonic type, 9
    mixed type, 9
    myths about, 13–17
    parts of body affected by, 9–10
    spastic type, 8
Cerebral spinal fluid, 6
Charities, 178

211

Cheated, feeling, 20–21
Child abuse, 7
Children's hospital, 26
Children's Justice Act, 45
Children with Disability Temporary Care Reauthorization Act, 45
Children with Special Health Care Needs, 178
Choices, making, 106–107, 148
Church youth groups, 146
Cleanliness, 100–101, 164
Clonus, 184
Cognition, 61–62
Cognitive milestones, 63t
Communication, 105, 136–139
Communication boards, 138
Community integration, 171–172
Community rehabilitation centers, 26
Competitive employment, 160
Comprehensive evaluations, 115–116
Computers, 142
Conferences, 94
Confusion, 19
Constipation, 70
Contractures, 58
Contributions to society, 154–156
Convulsions, 68
Cortical visual impairment, 72
Counseling, 28–29
Cytomegalovirus, 6

Day care, 45–46
Deinstitutionalization, 174
Delivery complications, 7
Denial, 19–20
Dental problems, 73
Development
　mental, 61–64
　normal, 53–55t
　physical, 56–60
　social, 65–67
Developmental Disabilities, Dept. of, 177
Developmental pediatrician, 78
Digestive problems, 69
Diplegia, 10, 89

Discipline, 104–107
Dislocation, 58
Divorce rates, 34
Dressing, 100
Drowning, 7
Due process, 114
Dyskinesia, 9
Dystonia, 9

Early intervention, 27, 49, 110, 117–120
Eating problems, 69, 74–76, 99, 101
Education
　legislation, 109–111t
　mainstreaming and inclusion, 130–132
　regular and special, 121–123
　sex, 163–166
　team, 128–129
　vocational, 159
Education, Dept. of, 114, 177
Education for All Handicapped Children Act (EHA), 109–110
Education of the Handicapped Act Amendments of 1986, 110, 117
Electrical stimulation, 85
Electrocution, 7
Elementary and Secondary Education Act Amendments, 109
Emotions
　acceptance, 22
　anger, 21
　bargaining, 21
　confusion, 19
　denial, 19–20
　feeling cheated, 20–21
　guilt, 20
Employment, 159
　competitive, 160
　resources for, 162
　sheltered workshop, 161
　supported, 160–161
　work activity center/adult day care, 161
Empowerment home, 107
Encephalitis, 6
Equipment, 176

# INDEX

Estate planning, 180
*Exceptional Parent Magazine*, 27
Expectations, 88–91
Exploration of environment, 66–67

Falls, 71
Family, 23–25
Family-centered service, 120
Family unit, 117
Fear, 35
Feeding problems, 3, 74–76, 185
Finances, 51, 175–178
Financial planning, 179–181
Floppy child, 4, 9
Free appropriate public education, 109
Freedom of Information Act, 165
Friends, 23–25, 145–147
Frustration, 64, 105

Gastroenterologist, 78
Gastroesophageal reflux, 69
Gastrostomy tube, 75
Genetic disorders, 7
German measles, 6
Glossary, 186–191
Goals, 124–127
    realistic, 151–153
Government agencies, 177–178
Grandparents, 42–43
Grants, 178
Grieving patterns, 23
Group homes, 174
Guardianship, 181
Guilt, 20

Habilitation, 127
Habilitation training, 102–103
Head injuries, 7
Health and Human Services, Dept. of, 27, 177
Healthcare team, 77–79
Health Department, 49
Health problems, 68–71
Hearing impairments, 72–73
Helmets, 71
Hemiplegia, 10, 89
Herpes, 6

Hip dislocation, 58
Hippotherapy, 81
Hobbies. *See* Interests
Home care, 15, 102–103
Home care aide, 103
Housing, 171–174
Hydrocephalus, 69
Hyperthermia, 7
Hypertonia, 8
Hypothermia, 7
Hypotonic cerebral palsy, 9, 89

Improvement, 14–15
Inclusion, 122–123, 131–132
Independence, fostering, 99–101
Independent living, 172
Individualized education program (IEP), 110, 112–113, 125–128, 158
Individualized family services plan (IFSP), 110, 118, 124–125, 157
Individualized habilitation plan (IHP), 103, 127
Individuals with Disabilities Education Act (IDEA), 110, 121, 158
Infant evaluations, 116
Infection, 6
Information, need for, 11–12
Inherited disorder, 13–14
Inhibitive cast/splint, 84
Insurance, 176–177
Intelligence tests, 62
Interaction with others, 67
Interdisciplinary team, 115
Interests, developing, 148–150
Intermediate care facilities, 174

Jewel, Gerry, 154–155
Job coach, 160
Joints, 58

Kyphosis, 58

Labor complications, 7
Laminectomy, 84
Language, 137
Learning, 133–135

213

Learning disability, 61
Least restrictive environment, 109
Letter of medical necessity, 176
Letting go, 182–183
Licensed practical nurse, 79
Lifting, 50
Limp baby, 4
Living arrangements, 171
　group homes, 174
　independent living, 172
　residential settings, 174
　semi-independent living, 172
　shared living, 173
　special foster care, 172

Magazines, list of, 196–197
Mainstreaming, 122–123, 130–132
Manipulation, 107
Marriage
　and cerebral palsy, 168–169
　parental, nurturing, 34–36
Masturbation, 163
Mediation, 113
Medicaid, 177
Medicare, 177
Medication, behavioral, 107
Meetings, 94
Meningitis, 6
Menstruation, 164
Mental development, 61–64
Mental retardation, 14, 61
Mentor, 149
Microcephaly, 6
Milestones, 55t, 63t, 116
Mixed cerebral palsy, 9
Monoplegia, 10
Mother's United for Moral Support, 27
Motor skills, 56–57
Motor vehicle accidents, 7
Movement problems, 3
Multidisciplinary evaluation, 115
Muscles, 57–58
Music therapy, 81
Myths about cerebral palsy, 13–17

Nasogastric tube, 75
National Father's Network, 27

National Information Center for Children and Youth with Disabilities, 27, 114
Negative behavior, 105
Negative talk, 31–32
Neonatologist, 77
Neurodevelopmental therapist, 81
Neurodevelopmental treatment, 81
Neurological problems, 68
Neurologist, 78
Neuropsychologist, 78
Neurosurgeon, 78
Newsletters, list of, 196–197
Nonnutrive sucking, 75
Normal development, 53–55t
Nurse, 79, 118–119
Nurse's aide, 79

Object permanence, 62
Occupational therapist, 79–80, 118
Oral motor coordination, 74
Oral motor therapy, 74–75
Organization, 92–95
Orogastric tube, 75
Orthopedic problems, 69
Orthopedic surgery, 85
Orthopedist, 60, 78
Orthotics, 85
Osteotomy, 60
Other parents, 26–27
Overweight, 69
Overwhelmed, feelings of being, 19
Oxygen, lack of, 6

Pain, 16
Parental rights, 112–114
Parenthood, 34
　and cerebral palsy, 169–170
Parent Training and Information Centers, 114
Pediatrician, 78
Peristalsis, 69
Personal care attendant, 79, 103
Physiatrist, 78
Physical development
　bones, 58
　joints, 58

# INDEX

motor skills, 56–57
muscles, 57–58
prevention of problems, 58–60
Physical education, 184
Physical medicine physician, 78
Physical therapist, 79–80, 118–119
Physical therapy assistant, 79
Pity, 32, 107
Play, 67, 96–98
Pneumonia, 70
Poisoning, 7
Positioning, of body, 100, 136, 192–193
Positive contributions, 154–156
Pregnancy complications, 7
Prevention and blame, 16–17
Primary service provider, 77, 118–119
Privacy, lack of, 34
Privileges, withholding, 106
Problem behaviors, 104–107
Professional support, 28–29
Psychiatrist, 78
Psychologist, 78, 118
Puberty, 164
Public library, 27
Punishments, 106

Quadriplegia, 10, 89

Recognition of family, 16
Recreation therapy, 81
Reeve, Christopher, 154
Registered nurse, 79, 118–119
Regular education, 121–123
Rehabilitation, 102
Rehabilitation Act, 123
Rehabilitation Engineering and Assistive Technology Society of North America, 176
Replacement child, 47–48
Residential settings, 174
Resource room, 122
Resources, list of, 198–204
Respecting child's personality, 33
Respite care, 44–45, 50, 95
Rewards, 106
Rh incompatibility, 6–7

Rights and responsibilities, 94
Rubella, 6

School attendance, 15
Scoliosis, 58
Scouting, 146, 149
Second baby, 47–48
Seizure medications, 68
Seizures, 68
Selective dorsal rhizotomy, 84
Self-care, 100
Self-injurious behaviors, 104
Self-stimulating behaviors, 67, 90, 104
Semi-independent living, 172
Sensory integration, 81
Sensory integration therapist, 81
Sensory overload, 105
Sex education, 163–166
Sexual abuse, 165
Sexuality, 167–168
Shared living, 173
Sheltered workshop, 161
Siblings, 37–41
Sibling Support Project, 27
Sign language, 138
Single-parent family, 49–51
Sisters, 37–41
Skin problems, 71
Small brain, 6
Social development, 65–67
Socialization, 145–147
Social Security Administration, 177–178
Societal contributions, 154–156
Spastic cerebral palsy, 8
Spasticity, 8
Special education, 26, 110, 121–123
Special education teacher, 121–122
Special foster care, 172
Special needs trust, 180
Specialness of all family members, 31–33
Special Olympics, 146
Speech pathologist, 79–80, 118–119
Spinal stabilization, 60
Splints, 84, 184
Sports, adapted, 146

Spouses, 34–36
State Rehabilitation Commissions, 27
Static encephalopathy, 5
Sterilization, 169
Strabismus, 72
Strangers, 23–25
Strengths, 155
Stress, 35
Stridor, 70
Subluxation, 58
Suffocation, 7
Supplemental Security Income (SSI), 177–178
Supported employment, 160–161
Support groups, 27
Swallow function study, 75, 185
Switch, adapted, 141–142
Symbols, 138

Tantrums, 106
Technical Assistance for Parent Programs (TAPP), 114
Teenagers, 67, 166
Teeth, 73
Tenotomy, 60
Tetracycline, 73
Therapy, 80–82, 185
Toddler evaluations, 116
Toys, adaptive, 96–98, 140–141
Tracheostomy, 70
Transdisciplinary team, 118
Transition plan, 126–127, 157–158
Traveling, 149
Trends in medical management, 83–86
Triggers for problem behaviors, 104–105
Triplets, 41
Tube feedings, 75
Twins, 41

Urinary tract infections, 71
Urologist, 78

Ventilator, 70
Ventricles, 6
Vision problems, 72
Visual field deficit, 72
Vocational education, 159
Vocational Rehabilitation, Dept. of, 177

Wheelchair, 141–142, 185
Work activity center, 161
Working, 159–162